MODERN NUTRITION
Edited by Ira Wolinsky and James F. Hickson, Jr.

Published Titles
Manganese in Health and Disease, Dorothy Klimis-Tavantzis
Nutrition and AIDS: Effects and Treatment, Ronald R. Watson
*Nutrition Care for HIV Positive Persons: A Manual for Individuals
    and Their Caregivers*, Saroj M. Bahl and James F. Hickson, Jr.
Calcium and Phosphorus in Health and Disease, John J. B. Anderson and
    Sanford C. Garner

Edited by Ira Wolinsky

Published Titles
Practical Handbook of Nutrition in Clinical Practice, Donald F. Kirby and
    Stanley J. Dudrick
Handbook of Dairy Foods and Nutrition, Gregory D. Miller, Judith K. Jarvis and
    Lois D. McBean
Advanced Nutrition: Macronutrients, Carolyn D. Berdanier
Childhood Nutrition, Fima Lifshitz
Antioxidants and Disease Prevention, Harinder S. Garewal
Nutrition and Cancer Prevention, Ronald R. Watson and Siraj I. Mufti
Nutrition and Health: Topics and Controversies, Felix Bronner
Nutritional Concerns of Women, Ira Wolinsky and Dorothy Klimis-Tavantzis
Nutrients and Gene Expression: Clinical Aspects, Carolyn D. Berdanier
Advanced Nutrition: Micronutrients, Carolyn D. Berdanier
Nutrition and Women's Cancer, Barbara C. Pence and Dale M. Dunn

Forthcoming Titles
Laboratory Tests for the Assessment of Nutritional Status, 2nd Edition,
    H. E. Sauberlich
Nutrition: Chemistry and Biology, 2nd Edition, Julian E. Spallholz,
    L. Mallory Boylan and Judy A. Driskell
Child Nutrition: An International Perspective, Noel W. Solomons
Handbook of Nutrition for Vegetarians, Rosemary A. Ratzin
Melatonin in the Promotion of Health, Ronald R. Watson
Nutrition and the Eye, Allen Taylor
Advanced Human Nutrition, Denis Medeiros and Robert E. C. Wildman
Nutrients and Foods in AIDS, Ronald R. Watson

NUTRITION & WOMEN'S CANCERS

BARBARA C. PENCE, Ph.D.
DALE M. DUNN, M.D.

CRC Press
Boca Raton Boston London New York Washington, D.C.

Library of Congress Cataloging-in-Publication Data

Catalog information may be obtained from the Library of Congress.

This book contains information obtained from authentic and highly regarded sources. Reprinted material is quoted with permission, and sources are indicated. A wide variety of references are listed. Reasonable efforts have been made to publish reliable data and information, but the author and the publisher cannot assume responsibility for the validity of all materials or for the consequences of their use.

Neither this book nor any part may be reproduced or transmitted in any form or by any means, electronic or mechanical, including photocopying, microfilming, and recording, or by any information storage or retrieval system, without prior permission in writing from the publisher.

The consent of CRC Press LLC does not extend to copying for general distribution, for promotion, for creating new works, or for resale. Specific permission must be obtained in writing from CRC Press LLC for such copying.

Direct all inquiries to CRC Press LLC, 2000 Corporate Blvd., N.W., Boca Raton, Florida 33431.

E56-50

Trademark Notice: Product or corporate names may be trademarks or registered trademarks, and are used only for identification and explanation, without intent to infringe.

© 1998 by CRC Press LLC

No claim to original U.S. Government works
International Standard Book Number 0-8493-8562-8
Printed in the United States of America 1 2 3 4 5 6 7 8 9 0
Printed on acid-free paper

TABLE OF CONTENTS

SERIES PREFACE FOR MODERN NUTRITION

The CRC Series in Modern Nutrition is dedicated to providing the widest possible coverage of topics in nutrition. Nutrition is an interdisciplinary, interprofessional field par excellence. It is noted by its broad range and diversity. We trust the titles and authorship in this series will reflect that range and diversity.

Published for a scholarly audience, the volumes in the CRC Series in Modern Nutrition are designed to explain, review, and explore present knowledge and recent trends, developments, and advances in nutrition. As such, they will also appeal to the educated layman. The format for the series will vary with the needs of the author and the topic, including, but not limited to, edited volumes, monographs, handbooks, and texts.

Contributors from any bona fide area of nutrition, including the controversial, are welcome.

Ira Wolinsky, Ph.D.
Series Editor

PREFACE

This book was undertaken in an effort to integrate what we know about nutrition and prevention of cancers that occur predominantly in women. In the past 20 years much has been published about the role of nutrition and dietary factors in many cancers, but there was a need to integrate all of the nutritional epidemiology with what else was known about the genetics and epidemiology of cancers in women. The cancers chosen for this analysis are those which occur only or predominantly in women, including breast, cervical, endometrial, and ovarian cancer, as well as those that also occur in men but which are seen in a very high incidence in women, such as cancer of the lung and colon. We have provided an introductory chapter on general methodologies associated with the field of nutrition and cancer. In each subsequent chapter and for each tumor type, we describe the general pathology of the disease, the genetics, general epidemiological factors, and finally, provide a review of the important dietary factors that have been studied in relation to the specific disease. Each chapter is summarized as to findings and recommendations. Finally, we briefly discuss women's cancer issues from a national policy standpoint with a review of current large clinical trials involving diet and cancer prevention in women. The final chapter provides an overview and recommendations for further research in the field of nutrition and female cancer. As the discipline of molecular biology becomes a ubiquitous technique in all areas of cancer research, including nutritional epidemiology, it is apparent that diet and genetics must be considered in an integrated fashion in order to evaluate the contributions of each.

Barbara C. Pence
Dale M. Dunn

ABOUT THE AUTHORS

Barbara Constable Pence, Ph.D., is Professor of Pathology at Texas Tech University Health Sciences Center School of Medicine in Lubbock, Texas. She obtained a B.A. and subsequently an M.S. in the Department of Biological Sciences at Texas Tech University and her Ph.D. in Nutrition and Experimental Pathology, also at Texas Tech. She was a Postdoctoral Fellow in Carcinogenesis at the M.D. Anderson Cancer Center/Science Park in Smithville, Texas. In 1987 she returned to Texas Tech to join the Department of Pathology at the Health Sciences Center as an Assistant Professor and achieved the rank of Professor in 1996. She is the Director of Research for the Department of Pathology, as well as Liaison Director for the West Texas Cancer Prevention Partnership, a rural mammography outreach program. Her research interests include the nutritional chemoprevention of colon and skin cancer and the interaction of nutrition and genetic damage. Her research has been supported by the National Cancer Institute, the American Institute for Cancer Research, and the Texas Cancer Council. She has published over 55 scientific articles and is a member of a number of federal and private grant review panels.

Dale Michael Dunn, M.D., is Professor and Chair of the Department of Pathology, as well as Regional Dean for the Lubbock campus, of the Texas Tech University School of Medicine. He obtained his B.S. at the University of Windsor, Windsor, Ontario, and his M.D. at the University of Western Ontario. He was trained in anatomic pathology at Maricopa County General Hospital, Phoenix, Arizona, and completed his training in both anatomic and clinical pathology at Baylor University Medical Center in Dallas, Texas. He has been on the faculty in the Department of Pathology at Texas Tech since 1984. During this time, in spite of his heavy administrative responsibilities, he has been actively involved in experimental cancer research, especially in gastrointestinal cancer prevention. In addition to numerous publications, he is also the recipient of several teaching awards.

CHAPTER 1

GENERAL EPIDEMIOLOGICAL METHODS RELEVANT TO NUTRITION AND CANCER IN WOMEN

CONTENTS

I. INTRODUCTION TO NUTRITIONAL EPIDEMIOLOGY

Many investigators have examined the impact of diet and nutrition on both total cancer incidence and mortality. These results are based upon evaluating the relationship between dietary factors and the observed cancer risk, migrant studies in which there are definite shifts in site-specific cancer rates among those people migrating to the United States, and supportive evidence from animal studies, as well as the biological relevance of diet to a particular type of cancer.[1] In 1981, Doll and Peto[2] estimated that 35% of all cancer mortality in the United States was related to diet, and previously Wynder and Gori[3] had estimated that nearly 40% of cancers among women are related to diet. Although it is not possible to quantify the contribution of diet to cancer risk for a particular site, it is sufficient to say that, excluding colon cancer, which is not specific to women, there appears to be a significant role for diet and nutrition in the etiology of most women's cancers. In this book, the role of nutrition in the potential causation of those cancers specific to or most prevalent in women will be discussed by site and by nutrient class. For the purposes of this discussion, those cancers included are lung, colorectal, breast, cervical, endometrial, and ovarian.

Nutritional epidemiology is a field of general epidemiology that is unique unto itself in terms of methods used to obtain data, the biases involved, and the degree of inference that can be extrapolated from the information compiled. In addition to epidemiological studies of nutrition and cancer, there are also *in vitro* studies and animal experiments, none of which will be a focus of this book. Indeed, a separate volume could be written on the amount of laboratory data alone in the area of nutrition and women's cancer. It is the purpose of this volume to limit our discussion to those human studies of diet, nutrition, and cancer which relate to the cancers we have chosen to examine.

II. TYPES OF FOOD CONSUMPTION DATA

Most studies of diet and cancer in populations use some type of food or nutrient consumption data to make comparisons between groups of varying risk for the particular type of cancer being studied. Three general approaches have been used to assess dietary information about the intake of certain foods or nutrients.[4] Because these methods profoundly influence the interpretation of the data on nutrition and cancer, their individual limitations will also be discussed.

A. Short-Term Recall/Diet Records

The first method to be discussed is the short-term recall and diet records type of dietary assessment. One commonly used method is the 24-hour recall, in which subjects are asked to report their food intake during the previous day. It has been the most widely used dietary assessment method in nutritional epidemiology.[4] Interviews are conducted by nutritionists or trained interviewers, often using visual aids such as food models or shapes to obtain data on the quantities of food consumed.[4] The 24-hour recall requires only 10–20 minutes to complete. The validity of the 24-hour recall has been assessed by observing the actual intake of subjects in a controlled environment and then interviewing them the following day. In such a validation study, Karvetti and Knuts[5] have observed that subjects both erroneously recalled foods that were not actually eaten and omitted foods that were consumed. The correlations they obtained

Coventry University
Lanchester Library
Tel 02476 887575

Borrowed Items 23/10/2010 17:07
XXXXXXXXXX4206

Item Title	Due Date
38001002078446	
* Nutrition and cancer preven	13/11/2010
38001002518847	
* Nutrition & women's cancer	13/11/2010

* Indicates items borrowed today
Thankyou

www.coventry.ac.uk

between nutrients calculated from the recalled information and what was eaten ranged from 0.58 to 0.74. Another study performed similarly found correlations between 0.28 and 0.87.[6] The most serious limitation of the 24-hour recall method is that dietary intake is highly variable from day to day.[4] Diet records can reduce the issue of day-to-day variation.

Diet records or food diaries are detailed meal-by-meal recordings of types and quantities of foods consumed during a specified period, such as 3–7 days.[4] In the ideal situation, subjects would weigh each portion of food before eating, or alternatively, household measures can be used to estimate portion sizes.[4] One problem with this method is that it requires considerable responsibility on the part of the subject, as well as a certain level of literacy and motivation. In fact, a bias that can result from this method is that the subject will become more acutely aware of what she is eating and self-induce an alteration in the diet. However, diet records do have the advantage of not being dependent on the subject's memory and do allow for the direct measurement of portion sizes. Although diet records can reduce the problem of day-to-day variability because the data are averaged out over the number of days for which data are taken, there is still the problem that only the most commonly eaten foods will be recorded.

The major criticism of the diet record/24-hour recall type of data is that they will only provide information on the current diet,[4] which makes them inappropriate for most case-control studies because the relevant exposure will have occurred earlier, and the diet may have changed as a result of the cancer or its treatment.[4] Although these types of data instruments could be used in prospective studies of diet and cancer, the sample size required for these studies would make the acquisition of this type of data prohibitive. In summary, the short-term and diet record methods of dietary assessment are generally expensive, unrepresentative of usual intake, and inappropriate for assessment of past diet.[4]

B. Food Frequency Questionnaire

A second type of dietary assessment used in studies of diet and cancer is the food frequency questionnaire (FFQ). This type of assessment has been developed and refined since the 1950s so that those in use today can yield data that are considerably more interpretable. The basic FFQ consists of two components: a food list and a frequency response section for subjects to report how often each food was eaten.[4] Since diets tend to be reasonably correlated from year to year, most questionnaires are designed to answer the questions in regard to diet for the preceding year. This also provides an entire range of seasons, so that the responses can be independent of time of year.[4] A multiple-choice format is usually chosen (five to ten choices), or in the case of the Block et al. FFQ,[7] the answers are requested in terms of frequency per day, week, or month. Portions are estimated by using either a description, a picture, or food models. However, some investigators have determined that portion size is relatively unimportant compared to the frequency of use.[8,9] In recent years, a number of culturally specific FFQs have been developed, thus allowing more accurate assessment of diet and cancer in multiethnic populations. In summary, the FFQ is a very practical epidemiological tool in diet and cancer investigations because it is easy to administer and process (usually by computer), and it yields reasonably reliable data. These attributes allow the feasible investigation of thousands of study subjects.

The interpretation of the epidemiological data on diet and cancer depends directly on the validity of the methods used to measure dietary intake.[4] During the past 10 years, a number of investigators have examined the validity of the FFQ, the most commonly used dietary assessment method in epidemiologic studies. Many have used the ability to correlate data from the FFQ with a biochemical indicator, such as plasma levels of certain nutrient classes, to quantitate validity of the questionnaire. Another method used to validate questionnaires is the comparison of computed intakes of nutrients with those based on other dietary assessment methods.[4] Although the degree of measurement error associated with nutrient intakes estimated from FFQs appears to be similar to that for many other epidemiological measures, these errors can lead to important underestimates of relative risks.[4] However, the validation studies have shown that the important associations will generally not be missed,[10] but that sample sizes would need to be several times larger than estimated if this measurement error did not exist.[11]

C. Biochemical Indicators of Diet

The third type of dietary assessment is biochemical indicators of diet. These are biochemical measurements made on blood and are often used to represent the intake of certain nutrients. The use of these methods has two advantages: the data do not depend on the memory or knowledge of the subject being evaluated, and the studies can be done retrospectively on stored blood specimens.[4] However, this latter advantage has also come under criticism due to the deterioration of some nutrients during long-term storage. Most commonly, blood serum or plasma has been used in epidemiologic studies, although some have examined subcutaneous fat, hair, and nails. The limitations of the use of biochemical indicators of nutrient intake are the high degree to which some of these nutrient levels are regulated in the plasma, their fluctuation over time, and the adverse effect of cancer itself on the levels of certain nutrients in the plasma or serum.

As a final note, a number of the studies discussed in this book will deal with energy balance, which is usually assessed by measurements of body dimensions and composition rather than direct measurement of the difference between energy intake and expenditure. The most commonly used anthropometric measurements are the Quetelet Index or the body mass index (weight divided by the second power of height). Sometimes relative weight or weight standardized for height is used. The major limitation of obesity estimates based on height and weight is that assessment of weight cannot differentiate between fat and lean body mass.[4] The use of skinfold thickness does not appear to be any more accurate than weight and height but can provide additional information on the distribution of body fat.[4] The ratio of waist-to-hip circumference also provides information on the distribution of body fat and has been used extensively to compare central fat distributions with peripheral fat distributions in regard to many diseases, including the hormonally sensitive cancers.[4] Height alone as a measurement has not been used extensively because it can be altered by nutritional deprivation during development and also is primarily genetically determined, assuming nutrition has been adequate.[4]

III. CORRELATIONAL OR ECOLOGICAL EPIDEMIOLOGIC STUDIES

Our discussion of the types of epidemiologic studies encountered in this volume begins with the observational studies. The basic function of most epidemiologic research designs is to permit a fair, unbiased contrast to be made between a group with and a group without a risk factor or intervention.[12] The observational epidemiologic studies are fairly quick and easy to perform and are useful for hypothesis generation.[12] However, they do not allow for hypothesis testing nor for causal conclusions to be drawn.[12] Until recently, most studies of diet and cancer were of the ecological or correlational study design. Ecologic studies generally compared the disease rates in populations with the population per capita consumption of specific dietary factors.[4] Often, the studies used "food disappearance" data, meaning that the dietary information in the study was based on national figures for food produced and imported minus the food that is exported.[4] International correlational studies that examine the relationships between diet and cancer have several advantages. Often the contrasts in intake are very large, such as are seen in the studies of fat consumption among different countries.[4] Additionally, the average diet is likely to become more stable over time, and the cancer rates for a large population are subject to fewer random errors than in smaller studies.[4]

However, there are a number of serious limitations to the use of correlational studies. One of the primary problems is that many of the potential determinants of cancer, besides the dietary factor of interest, may vary significantly within a population, and this will not be pulled out in the correlational study design. These variables might include genetic variability, other dietary factors, and other environmental or lifestyle influences.[4] Most correlational studies are also limited by the use of disappearance data that are only indirectly related to intake. As such, the aggregate data for a geographical unit as a whole may only be weakly related to the diets of those individuals in the population with the highest risk of the disease.[4] Another limitation of the international correlation studies is that they cannot be independently reproduced,[4] which is to say that the populations and their diets will tend to remain the same over time, and even reexamination of the data will not typically yield independent results for comparisons between studies. Taken together, these types of studies have been considered the weakest forms of evidence, although they have been extremely valuable in providing hypotheses to test relating diet and cancer.

Among the most valuable of the correlational studies are those of special exposure groups and the studies of migrant populations. Subgroups within a population that consume an unusual diet provide unique opportunities to study the relationship between consumption of specific dietary factors and diseases such as cancer. These subpopulations generally live within the same environment as a comparison group but, due to ethnic or religious considerations, may have significantly different diets. Much of what we have learned about diet and colon cancer in the early years of nutritional epidemiology came from studies of Seventh-Day Adventists, who were largely vegetarian and had half the expected rate of colon cancer.[13] Migrant studies have been particularly important in addressing the contribution of genetic factors to those results obtained in ecologic studies. It has been established for most cancers that populations migrating from an area with a characteristic cancer incidence pattern acquire the incidence rates of the new location. Thus, the genetic contribution remains constant, and the situation permits epidemiologists to examine the effects of a new environment and diet on the incidence of common cancers. This type of study design has been helpful in allowing us to understand how the high-fat Western diet can impact the rate of colon, breast, and prostate cancer.[14] Another type of ecological study that has been a significant contributor to our understanding of diet and cancer is the study of diet at different points in time within the same population. This type of design can determine the emergence of environmental factors responsible for changes in cancer incidence rates within a genetically similar group of people.[4]

IV. COHORT STUDIES: RETROSPECTIVE AND PROSPECTIVE

A cohort is a clearly identified group of people to be studied.[12] In cohort studies, investigators begin by assembling one or more cohorts, either by choosing persons specifically because they were or were not exposed to one or more risk factors to be studied or by taking a random sampling of the population.[12] There are two general types of cohort study: the prospective type and the retrospective type. In a prospective cohort study, the investigator assembles the study groups in the present time, collects baseline data on them, and continues to collect data over time.[12] There are a number of advantages to the prospective cohort study: the investigator is able to control the data collection as the study progresses, the risk estimates obtained are true risks for the groups studied, and many different disease outcomes can be studied, including some that were not anticipated at the beginning of the study.[12] However, there are also disadvantages, such as the limitation of the study to those risk factors which are defined at the inception of the study and, of course, the high cost and long wait for results. Retrospective studies can alleviate some of the time and cost problems associated with the prospective cohort study. In this approach, the investigator goes back in history to define a risk group and follows the members of the cohort to see what outcomes have occurred. Many diet and cancer studies utilize both types of cohort studies for data acquisition. The prospective cohort study, such as used in the Nurses' Health Study,[15-18] appears to be almost the gold standard for assessing the relationship between diet and cancer outcome, as we shall see in the numerous publications that have emanated from that study in all the subsequent chapters in this book.

V. CASE-CONTROL STUDIES

The investigator in a case-control study selects the case group on the basis of the outcome (i.e., having the disease of interest, such as cancer of a certain site, vs. not having the disease of interest) and compares the groups in terms of their frequency of past exposure to possible risk factors.[12] This type of design is used extensively in diet and cancer studies and has provided much of the most conclusive evidence we have, along with cohort studies, on dietary factors and cancer risk. Although these types of studies compare the risk of having the factor or dietary exposure between the two groups, the actual risk of the outcome cannot be determined from case-control studies because the underlying population is not known.[12] However, an estimate of the relative risk of the outcome (i.e., the cancer), called the odds ratio, can be determined in case-control studies.[12] In these studies, the cases and their matched controls (sometimes hospital based, but also community based) are assembled, and then they are questioned about the exposure of interest. These have been called retrospective studies for this reason.

Case-control studies are useful when a study must be done quickly, as opposed to a prospective cohort study, and inexpensively, although many risk factors may be considered in case-control studies, such as is the case with the use of the FFQ. Despite these obvious advantages, there are some drawbacks to the use of the case-control study design. A major problem is the potential for recall bias, which may be substantial in the case of a devastating disease such as cancer. People who experience an adverse event, such as breast cancer, may cogitate more about why the event might have happened and, therefore, may be more likely to recall previous risk factors than the people who have never experienced the event. This type of bias can also occur in dietary assessment in cases vs. controls, especially if the cases attribute more weight to certain perceived risk factors associated with their disease. Another problem with case-control studies is that it is not easy to know what the correct control group should be.[12] The controls are usually matched individually to the cases on the basis of age, sex, and often race. But where these controls come from can often lead to different results, such as the choice of other patients without the disease or healthy controls from the community. Often, the investigator may assemble two control groups, one of which is from the general population.[12]

VI. EXPERIMENTAL DESIGNS FOR HYPOTHESIS TESTING

The most rigorous evaluation of a dietary hypothesis is the randomized trial, optimally conducted as a double-blind experiment. In a randomized controlled clinical trial (RCCT), patients or subjects are enrolled in a study and then randomly assigned to one of the following groups: (1) the intervention group which will receive the experimental treatment or (2) the control group which will receive the nonexperimental treatment consisting of either a placebo (inert substance) or a standard method of treatment.[12] To be enrolled in an RCCT, the subjects must agree to participate without knowing whether they will be given the experimental or nonexperimental treatment. If possible, the observers who collect the data are also prevented from knowing which type of treatment each subject is given. When the study is done in this way so that neither participant nor observer knows which treatment is given, the trial is said to be a double-blind study.[12] To have true blinding, the placebo treatment should appear identical to the experimental treatment. This type of study design has been used successfully in the Physicians' Health Study[19] and is in use in the trials described in Chapter 8.

The principal strength of the RCCT is that potentially distorting variables should be distributed randomly between the treatment and control groups, thus minimizing confounding by these extraneous variables.[4] Experimental trials have been used to test a number of hypotheses that certain minor components of the diet can prevent cancer, especially since these nutrients can be easily formulated into pills and capsules. However, there are certain limitations to the use of the RCCT design in studies of diet and cancer. The time between the intervention and the emergence of the cancer of interest can be quite uncertain.[4] Compliance of the subjects for the intervention may be a problem, especially if the intervention requires a substantial change in dietary habits, such as changing to a low-fat diet or consuming significantly more fruits and vegetables than usual. Another potential limitation of these trials is the selection bias which occurs because the participants who enroll in such studies tend to be highly motivated and more health conscious.[4] This could be a serious bias to the results, in that those who may benefit from the intervention the most may not be participants because of their low enthusiasm for such activities. However, a number of interventional trials in the field of diet and cancer have been successfully completed, and others are ongoing, although there are these potential pitfalls.

VII. STATISTICS COMMONLY USED IN STUDIES OF DIET AND CANCER

Throughout this book, we will be discussing a multitude of different types of studies to illustrate the conclusions that can be drawn from the wealth of data available on diet and women's cancers. Certain statistics will be used to assess the associations between specific dietary factors or biochemical measurements and cancer risk. A risk factor is defined as "a characteristic which, if present and active, clearly increases the probability of a particular disease (in our case, cancer) in a group of persons who have the factor compared to an otherwise similar group of persons who do not."[12] However, a risk factor is not a necessary or a sufficient cause of the disease. Assessment of risk in epidemiologic studies depends on the measurement of contrast. In cohort studies, the contrast is between the frequency of disease in persons exposed to a risk factor and the frequency of disease in persons not exposed to the risk factor, such as dietary variables of interest.[12] In case-control studies, the contrast is between the frequency of the risk factor in the cases with the disease and the frequency of the disease in the control subjects without the disease.

A. Relative Risk

Two commonly used statistics throughout this book are relative risk (RR) and odds ratio (OR). First, attributable risk should be defined. The risk difference between the risk in the exposed group and those unexposed is also known as the attributable risk because it is also an estimate of the total risk that can be attributable to the specific risk factor after all other known causes have been taken into account. The RR is expressed in terms of a risk ratio or the risk in the exposed group divided by the risk in the unexposed group. If the risks are the same, the RR will be 1.0. Calculation of the RR provides a straightforward way of showing in relative terms how much different the risks are for the exposed group.[12] Relative differences in risk can also be expressed in terms of the OR.

B. Odds Ratio

The OR is somewhat different from the RR in that the RR describes the risk of the disease in the exposed group, whereas the odds of getting the disease in the exposed group is expressed by the OR. If the risk of getting the disease from the exposure is relatively large, then the OR is not the same as the RR. The OR can be calculated from case-control studies, but the RR cannot. The RR is appropriately calculated from the prospective cohort study. However, for diseases that are of low risk in the population (less than 5%), the OR may be used as an estimate of the risk of the disease.[12] ORs are also used in logistic regression analyses, which are seen in many reports of epidemiologic studies.

Table 1.1 Epidemiologic Study Designs

Type of Study	Design	Risk Statistic
Correlational	Per capita consumption of specific dietary factors	r^a
Cohort	Choose persons based on exposure to risk factors	
Prospective	Assemble study group; follow over time	RR
Retrospective	Goes back in time to define a risk group to follow	RR
Case-control	Case group selected by having the disease of interest	OR

^{a} r = Pearson product-moment correlation coefficient.

However, a discussion of more complex epidemiologic statistics is beyond the scope of this chapter.

VIII. SUMMARY

In summary, there are a number of types of epidemiology study designs which will be studied in our assessment of diet, nutrition, and cancer in women (Table 1.1). For the most part, they will be of the cohort or case-control design, and therefore, we will be predominantly concerned with RRs and ORs in terms of comparisons among studies. These definitions are summarized in Table 1.1. It is hoped that the reader has benefited from this brief description of the methodology used in diet and cancer studies and that the concepts of selection and recall bias, confounding, and types of dietary assessment tools will allow better interpretation of the data and studies presented.

REFERENCES

1. Committee on Diet and Health, Food and Nutrition Board, Commission on Life Sciences, National Research Council, *Diet and Health: Implications for Reducing Chronic Disease Risk*, National Academy Press, Washington, D.C., 1989, chap. 22.
2. Doll, R. and Peto, R., The causes of cancer: quantitative estimates of avoidable risks in the United States today, *J. Natl. Cancer Inst.*, 66, 1191, 1981.
3. Wynder, E.L. and Gori, G.B., Contribution of the environment to cancer incidence: an epidemiological exercise, *J. Natl. Cancer Inst.*, 58, 825, 1977.
4. Willett, W.C., Diet and nutrition, in *Cancer Epidemiology and Prevention*, Schottenfeld, D. and Fraumeni, J.F., Jr., Eds., Oxford University Press, New York, 1996, chap. 21.
5. Karvetti, R.L. and Knuts, L.R., Validity of the 24-hour recall, *J. Am. Diet. Assoc.*, 85, 1437, 1985.

6. Madden, J.P., Goodman, S.J., and Guthrie, H.A., Validity of the 24-hour recall: analysis of data obtained from elderly subjects, *J. Am. Diet. Assoc.*, 68, 143, 1976.
7. Block, G., Hartman, A.M., Dresser, C.M., Carroll, M.D., Gannon, J., and Gardner, L., A data-based approach to diet questionnaire design and testing, *Am. J. Epidemiol.*, 124, 453, 1986.
8. Samet, J.M., Humble, C.G., and Skipper, B.E., Alternatives in the collection and analysis of food frequency interview data, *Am. J. Epidemiol.*, 120, 572, 1984.
9. Block, G., Woods, M., Potosky, A., and Clifford, C., Validation of a self-administered diet questionnaire using multiple diet records, *J. Clin. Epidemiol.*, 43, 1327, 1990.
10. Rosner, B., Willett, W.C., and Spiegelman, D., Correction of logistic regression relative risk estimates and confidence intervals for systematic within-person measurement error, *Stat. Med.*, 8, 1051, 1989.
11. Walker, A.M. and Blettner, M., Comparing imperfect measures of exposure, *Am. J. Epidemiol.*, 121, 783, 1985.
12. Jekel, J.F., Elmore, J.G., and Katz, D.L., *Epidemiology, Statistics, and Preventive Medicine*, W.B. Saunders, Philadelphia, 1996.
13. Phillips, R.L., Garfinkel, L., Kuzma, J.W., Beeson, W.L., Lotz, T., and Brin, B., Mortality among California Seventh-Day Adventists for selected cancer sites, *J. Natl. Cancer Inst.*, 65, 1097, 1980.
14. Cotran, R.S., Kumar, V., and Robbins, S.L., *Robbins Pathologic Basis of Disease*, 5th ed., W.B. Saunders, Philadelphia, 1994.
15. London, S.J., Colditz, G.A., Stampfer, M.J., Willett, W.C., Rosner, B., and Speizer, F.E., Prospective study of relative weight and breast cancer, *J. Am. Med. Assoc.*, 262, 2853, 1989.
16. Willett, W.C., Hunter, D.J., Stampfer, M.J., Colditz, G., Manson, J.E., Spiegelman, D., Rosner, B., Hennekens, C.H., and Speizer, F.E., Dietary fat and fiber in relation to risk of breast cancer, *J. Am. Med. Assoc.*, 268, 2037, 1992.
17. Hunter, D.J., Stampfer, M.J., Colditz, G.A., Manson, J., Rosner, B., Hennekens, C.H., Speizer, F.E., and Willett, W.C., A prospective study of consumption of vitamins A, C and E and breast cancer risk, *Am. J. Epidemiol.*, 134, 715, 1991.
18. Hunter, D.J., Morris, J.S., Stampfer, M.J., Colditz, G.A., Speizer, F.E., and Willett, W.C., A prospective study of selenium status and breast cancer risk, *J. Am. Med. Assoc.*, 264, 1128, 1990.
19. Hennekens, C.H., Buring, J.E., Manson, J.E., Stampfer, M., Rosner, B., Cook, N.R., Belanger, C., LaMotte, F., Gaziano, J.M., Ridker, P.M., Willett, W., and Peto, R., Lack of effect of long-term supplementation with beta carotene on the incidence of malignant neoplasms and cardiovascular disease, *New Engl. J. Med.*, 334, 1145, 1996.

CHAPTER 2

NUTRITION AND BREAST CANCER

CONTENTS

I. GENERAL PATHOLOGY AND STATISTICS

Breast cancer is the most common cancer among women worldwide and accounts for about 30% of all newly diagnosed cancers in women in the United States and 17% of cancer-related deaths.[1] In contrast, male breast cancer is rare compared to cancer of the female breast, with a ratio worldwide of 1:70 to 1:130.[2]

Approximately 99% of all malignant breast neoplasms are carcinomas, and nearly all carcinomas of the breast are adenocarcinomas. Carcinoma is slightly more common in the left breast than in the right breast. The location of carcinoma of the breast in its primary instance is upper/outer quadrant—50%, nipple and areolar area—20%, upper/inner quadrant—10%, lower/outer quadrant—10%, and lower/inner quadrant—10%.

A. Histologic Types and Incidences

According to the World Health Organization classification of female breast carcinoma, the following histological types are noted (adapted from WHO[3]):

  A. Noninvasive
     1a. Intraductal carcinoma
     1b. Intraductal carcinoma with Paget's disease
     2. Lobular carcinoma *in situ*
  B. Invasive (infiltrating)
     1a. Invasive ductal carcinoma—not otherwise specified
     1b. Invasive ductal carcinoma with Paget's disease
     2. Invasive lobular carcinoma
     3. Medullary carcinoma
     4. Colloid carcinoma (mucinous carcinoma)
     5. Tubular carcinoma

The incidences (%) of the various histologic types of invasive breast cancer are as follows (adapted from Fisher et al.[4]):

Invasive duct carcinoma	
Pure	52.6
Combined with other types	22.0
Medullary carcinoma	6.2
Colloid carcinoma	2.4
Paget's disease	2.3
Other pure types	2.0
Other combined types	1.6
Infiltrating lobular carcinoma	4.9
Combined lobular and ductal	6.0

Adenoid cystic carcinoma, apocrine carcinoma, and invasive papillary carcinoma are quite rare.

Intraductal carcinoma is a malignant solid tumor growth which occurs within a duct. Over 90% of breast carcinomas arise within ducts. They occur in the postmenopausal age group. The tumor consists of ducts filled with cellular cords with or without necrosis in the central portion of the tumor mass. Metastasis does not occur.

Papillary carcinoma is a malignancy of the duct system of the breast and consists of papillary epithelial structures. There is often a bloody discharge from the nipple. The microscopic appearance exhibits a papillary growth of epithelium, which exhibits atypical cells. Necrosis of the tumor tissue is not seen. This tumor can metastasize but generally causes more localized invasion and usually carries a better prognosis.

Infiltrating or invasive duct cell carcinoma is the most common and most studied type of carcinoma of the breast.[4] It is an adenocarcinoma, and it often forms a hard mass. The tumor forms a mass commonly 2–3 cm in maximum diameter. The tumor infiltrates adjacent tissue with a marked desmoplastic fibrosis of the stroma which compresses the tumor cells. The marked desmoplasia accounts for the oftentimes stony hardness of the tumor mass. Areas of calcification may be seen in those tumors with greater age, but the calcification tends to be small and punctate. The tumor cells are disposed in cords, solid cell nests, tubes, glands, anastomosing masses, and mixtures of all these. The tumor in two-thirds of cases exhibits lymph node metastasis.

Medullary carcinoma is a duct cell adenocarcinoma. The tumor forms a large soft mass in the breast. Microscopically, the tumor is formed of solid sheets of cells with vesicular and often pleomorphic nuclei, containing prominent nucleoli and frequent mitoses. A lymphocytic infiltrate is usually present between the neoplastic cell masses. As a rule, the more extensive the lymphocytic infiltration, the less aggressive the tumor. The lymph nodes are generally negative for metastasis in this condition.[5]

Mucinous (colloid) adenocarcinoma occurs in older women and grows slowly, producing a large, soft gelatinous tumor. Microscopically, there may be large pools of amorphous, pale blue mucin that dissect into surrounding tissue.

Paget's disease is a duct cell carcinoma which arises in the main excretory ducts of the breast beneath the nipple and extends to involve the skin of the nipple and areola. The condition can clinically appear like eczema of the nipple. It occurs generally in the postmenopausal female. Microscopically, the typical appearance of Paget's disease is that of central intraductal carcinoma beneath the nipple. There are large anaplastic cells with pale cytoplasm (Paget's cells) within the squamous epithelium surrounding the opening of the duct into the nipple.

Lobular carcinoma *in situ* arises in the female mammary lobule or in the terminal ductules in the mammary lobule. These lesions are often extremely difficult to differentiate from atypical lobular hyperplasia seen in fibrocystic disease.[6]

Infiltrating lobular carcinoma arises from the cells of the lobules and terminal ductules. In 20% of cases, there is bilateral involvement in the other breast. Microscopically, strands of tumor cells characteristically infiltrate in an "Indian file" manner. The cells are often uniform with little evidence of cytologic atypia.

Sarcoma of the female breast constitutes less than 1% of all breast neoplasms. Half are cystosarcoma phyllodes (fibroepithelial) more appropriately referred to as phylloides tumor. This can be either benign or malignant. Microscopically, the pattern is that of an intracanalicular fibroadenoma, but the stroma is more cellular than a fibroadenoma. The stroma of this lesion may undergo malignant transformation.

B. Clinical Staging of Breast Cancer

The following system of clinical staging has been adopted by most U.S. centers. The American Joint Committee on Cancer Staging divides the clinical stages as follows:[7]

Stage I	is a tumor less than 2 cm in diameter without nodal involvement and no metastases. (80% five-year survival)
Stage II	is a tumor less than 5 cm in diameter with involved but movable axillary nodes and no distant metastases or a tumor greater than 5 cm without nodal involvement or distant metastases. (65% five-year survival)
Stage III	is all breast cancers of any size with possible skin involvement, pectoral and chest fixation, and nodal involvement including axillary nodes, fixed but without disseminated metastases. (40% five-year survival)

Stage IV is any form of breast cancer with or without nodal involvement, pectoral fixation, skin ulceration, or chest wall fixation, but having disseminated metastases. (10% five-year survival) *

II. GENERAL EPIDEMIOLOGY OF BREAST CANCER

Before we discuss the lifestyle factors associated with risk for breast cancer, it seems appropriate to mention those risk factors inherent in a woman's body which are not really considered to be specifically genetic, nor are they easily defined as environmental, although they may have some indirect environmental causes. These would include the well-known risk factors included in the Gail model[8] of breast cancer risk, and these would be the reproductive factors: age at menarche, age at menopause, pregnancy, lactation, and menstrual cycle length. The Gail model has been used extensively to numerically determine a woman's individual risk, especially as an assessment tool for eligibility for participation in the Breast Cancer Prevention Trial using tamoxifen. Although this model seems appropriate for use in that study, it has come under criticism in recent years.

A. Reproductive Factors

Early age at menarche has been demonstrated as a risk factor for breast cancer in most case-control studies. In general, an approximately 20% decrease in breast cancer risk can be seen for each year that menarche is delayed.[9] Henderson et al.[10] examined this relationship using not the absolute age at onset of menses, but the age at which regular periods were established. For a fixed age at menarche, women who established regular menstrual cycles within 1 year of age of onset had more than double the risk of breast cancer than those who had a 5-year or longer delay in the onset of regular periods. Women with an early menarche (before age 12) and a rapid establishment of regular periods had a fourfold increase in breast cancer risk, compared with those women whose menarche was delayed past age 13 or longer.[9] Henderson et al.[11] further postulated that it is the regular ovulatory cycles that increase the risk of breast cancer because there are higher circulating levels of estrogen and progesterone,[12] and cumulative frequency of ovulatory cycles is an indicator of cumulative estrogen and progesterone exposure. Over the past 100 years, the average age at menarche in the United States has progressively decreased.[9] This has been shown to be directly related to childhood growth patterns,[13] since attainment of a critical body weight to height ratio appears to be necessary for menarche to occur. It seems that improved nutrition of children and control of infectious diseases have served to lower the age of menarche in the Western world and, along with it, to increase the risk of breast cancer.

* From Cotran, R.S., Kumar, V., and Robbins, S.L., *Robbins Pathologic Basis of Disease*, 5th ed., W.B. Saunders, Philadelphia, 1994, 1107. With permission.

Age at menopause is another reproductive factor associated with breast cancer risk. It has been estimated that women who experience natural menopause at age 45 or younger have only one-half the risk of women whose menopause occurs at age 55 or older.[9] Artificial menopause by either bilateral oophorectomy or pelvic irradiation also markedly reduces breast cancer risk.[9] It has also been shown that a unilateral oophorectomy or simple hysterectomy does not alter risk.[14]

One of the earliest known factors associated with breast cancer risk is the decreased risk associated with increased parity and the increased risk seen in single women.[9] It was first reported in 1970[15] that single and nulliparous women both had the same 1.4-fold increased risk of breast cancer compared to parous, married women. However, these authors demonstrated that the protective effect of this phenomenon was confined to a protective effect of early age at first birth. Women who had their first birth under age 20 had about half the risk of nulliparous women,[9] and subsequent births had no effect on risk for breast cancer. It was also found that married women who have a late full-term pregnancy actually have an elevated risk for breast cancer,[15] and this has apparently been confirmed repeatedly.[9] This is thought to be related to lowered prolactin levels in parous compared with nulliparous women[16] and higher levels of sex hormone binding globulin and lower levels of free estradiol than in nulliparous women.

The practice of lactation has also been linked to lower risk for breast cancer. This is not unexpected, because one of the effects of nursing is that it results in a substantial delay in the reestablishment of ovulation following a completed pregnancy.[9] Because most women do not nurse for extended periods of time, it has been difficult to accurately establish estimates of risk associated with lactation. However, a recent case-control study from China, where lactation is of long duration, concluded that there is a progressive reduction in breast cancer risk seen with an increasing number of years of lactation experience.[17]

Menstrual cycle length has also been considered as a risk factor for breast cancer, in keeping with an estrogenic stimulation hypothesis of etiology. In a retrospective study of average menstrual cycle length, it was reported that the average length of breast cancer patients was 26.4 days, while that of controls was 28.6 days.[18] This has been confirmed by La Vecchia et al.[19] and also in a study comparing the cycle length of Japanese women and U.S. women, with the Japanese women having longer cycles.[20] The relationship between shorter cycles and risk appears to be associated again with the cumulative frequency of ovulatory cycles and an increased estrogen exposure.[9]

B. Fibrocystic Disease

Another hormonally related factor which has been investigated in regard to breast cancer risk is the presence of benign fibrocystic breast disease. It was first reported in 1977 by Kodlin et al.[21] that women who have cystic breast disease have a two- to threefold increased risk of breast cancer. Black et al.[22] found that they could establish a subgroup of women with benign breast disease with "atypical" epithelial changes, and that these women had a fivefold increased risk of breast cancer, compared to other women with benign breast disease without "atypia." This association has been further researched,[23, 24] and these investigators have shown that there is little or no increased risk in women with nonproliferative breast disease, a modest increase in risk in women with proliferative disease without atypia, and a four- to fivefold increase in those with atypical hyperplasia. The relationship between atypical hyperplasia and breast cancer has been further confirmed by Ma and Boyd[25] in a meta-analysis of 18 studies published between 1960 and 1992. The pooled estimate from all studies examined gave an odds ratio of 3.67 for the association between atypical hyperplasia and breast cancer. This further supports the premise that atypical hyperplasia of the breast epithelium is a risk factor for breast cancer.

C. Nonreproductive Factors

1. Introduction

There are a number of nonreproductive lifestyle factors which have been examined for an association with risk for breast cancer. Among those most studied are oral contraceptive use, estrogen replacement therapy, breast implants, physical activity, cigarette smoking, and stress. Probably the most studied environmental risk factor, aside from diet, would be the use of oral contraceptives. There have been a number of studies on this subject since 1966 when their use became widespread. Hawley et al.[26] performed a meta-analysis of case-control studies of oral contraceptive use and breast cancer on published studies from 1966 to 1990. The categories of use were "ever oral contraceptive users," "long-term oral contraceptive users," and "oral contraceptive use before a first full-term pregnancy." For the first two categories of ever and long-term users, no association could be detected between oral contraceptive use and the development of breast cancer.[26] However, in the category of use before a first full-term pregnancy, a significant correlation was found. This meta-analysis suggested that there is a possible increased risk of breast cancer in women who use oral contraceptives before a first full-term pregnancy. However, these data must be cautiously interpreted in view of the data linking age at first pregnancy with breast cancer risk, in that if a woman postpones first pregnancy by taking oral contraceptives, this may only be a confounder for that association.

2. Hormone Replacement Therapy

The links between hormone replacement therapy (HRT) and cancers of both the breast and endometrium have been recently reviewed by Hulka.[27] A number of studies in the United States and Europe of HRT and breast cancer have been conducted,[27] and the relative risks generally range between 1.0 and 2.7, except for a study of women in Britain which reported relative risks between 3.6 and 5.3.[28] This is thought to be related to the source of hormones in Europe, where estradiol and synthetic estrogens are more common and seem to increase the risk somewhat.[27] Hulka[27] concludes that the risks from HRT are modest, with estimates generally in the range of 1.3–2.0, dependent on the duration of use and the recency of use before diagnosis. Long-term use appears to be a critical issue, although the magnitude of the duration effects is a relative risk of greater than 1.5 after 10–15 years of use. Adding progestins to the estrogen regimen may actually increase breast cancer risk, whereas this practice decreases risk of endometrial cancer. However, since progestins have only been in use for about 15 years in HRT, there are not currently available reliable data on this type of HRT.[27] It has also been observed that particular subgroups, such as those with family history, benign proliferative disease, or late natural menopause, may experience greater risk.[27] However, in all of these associations, the relative risks are less than 2.

3. Physical Activity

There have been various indirect indications that physical activity can reduce breast cancer risk.[29] Frisch et al.[30] reported in 1985 that strenuous exercise in adolescence is associated with reduced breast cancer risk later in life by possibly delaying menarche and reducing the frequency of ovulation, two risk factors we have alluded to already. Several other studies from Finland,[31,32] Shanghai,[33] and Turkey[34] have also examined the relationship between certain occupations and breast cancer, but either no association was seen or associations were weakened by allowance for socioeconomic class.[34] However, one case-control study from California focused specifically on physical activity and showed a strong protection associated with physical activity, with an odds ratio of 0.42 for women who reported 3.8 hours/week or more of physical activity.[35] A more recent study by D'Avanzo et al.[29] analyzed data from a large multicenter case-control study in Italy for the relationship between occupational and leisure-time physical activity and breast cancer risk. They found that after adjustment for major confounding factors including total caloric intake, the odds ratios were all reduced for quartiles of physical activity compared to the lowest. There was a significant P for trend. They concluded that 36% of breast cancer cases could be prevented by increasing physical activity to the highest level reported in the study.[29]

4. Cigarette Smoking

Cigarette smoking and risk for breast cancer is another lifestyle variable which has been extensively studied, but still remains controversial. In 1982, MacMahon et al.[36] reported a reduction in estrogen levels in women smokers during the luteal phase of the menstrual cycle. They proposed the radical hypothesis that smoking might reduce the risk of breast cancer. Baron[37] suggested that smoking produced an antiestrogenic effect, altering the risk of several estrogen-related diseases such as osteoporosis and endometrial cancer. The exact mechanism for this apparent antiestrogenic effect is unclear. However, in 1986, Hiatt and Fireman[38] proposed a contrasting hypothesis that tobacco smoke may have a direct carcinogenic effect on the breast which could outweigh the benefits of any possible antiestrogenic effect. Numerous other investigations have been published (for review see Palmer and Rosenberg[39]). There have also been two reports of an increased risk of breast cancer in nonsmoking women married to smokers compared with nonsmoking women married to nonsmokers.[40,41] However, Palmer and Rosenberg[39] concluded that it is unlikely that cigarette smoking has a net effect on reducing risk of breast cancer, as well as little evidence to suggest that cigarette smoking materially increases risk, although it certainly increases the morbidity and mortality for other diseases.

5. Emotional Stress

The relationship between emotional stress and the development of breast cancer is controversial, since systematic studies of the subject are scarce.[42] Only one study has investigated the effects of certain life events and disease-free survival after diagnosis of breast cancer.[43] These authors did not find any significantly increased risk of relapse of breast cancer in those women who reported severe life events. However, others have reported that psychotherapy with a positive twist may improve survival in breast cancer patients.[44] However, there do not appear to be any studies demonstrating an association between a stressful life and increased risk of developing breast cancer.

6. In Situ Carcinoma

The incidence of *in situ* carcinoma of the breast has increased roughly fivefold since the 1970s, a rise largely attributable to the increased use of mammography screening.[45] Longnecker et al.[45] have recently examined the risk factors for *in situ* breast cancer from two population-based case-control studies in Los Angeles women. They reported that, in general, risk factors for *in situ* breast cancer were similar to those for invasive disease in this population. In premenopausal women, however, the risk of *in situ* breast cancer decreased with increasing body mass index, whereas for invasive disease, body mass index was unrelated to risk. This is in apparent contrast to a number of studies discussed under dietary fat in the section below. Additionally, in postmenopausal women with a known age at menopause, the use of unopposed estrogen HRT was associated with increased risk of *in situ* disease,[45] and a similar difference was seen for combined HRT. The authors concluded that increased screening in HRT users could account for some of the association with *in situ* disease.

7. Induced Abortion

The question of whether induced abortion is associated with breast cancer risk, first posed in 1981 by Pike et al.,[46] has received new attention with the 1994 report by Daling et al.[47] that a history of induced abortion was associated with a 50% increase in breast cancer risk in women who had been pregnant at least once. Rookus and van Leeuwen[48] reviewed the literature and found that the overall results for the association between abortion and breast cancer risk are inconclusive, with a positive association seen in five studies, no association in six studies, and a negative association in the only cohort study. These authors reexamined the issue in a Dutch case-control study of the history of spontaneous or induced abortion and breast cancer. Their results found that among parous women, a history of induced abortion was associated with a 90% increased risk of breast cancer, with no association found among nulliparous women.[48] They did, however, also find that in studies of abortion and cancer risk, if studies are based on information from study subjects only, reporting bias was a real problem. With this consideration in mind, the data from all similar studies of this risk factor could be suspect, and no firm conclusions can be drawn.

8. New Paradigm for Prevention

Finally, while we are still discussing the nondietary risk factors for breast cancer, it should be stated that most models of risk for this cancer address risks that occur during adulthood, or at least from the age of menarche on, and usually concentrate on events that influence postmenopausal risk. A new slant on this assumption has been gaining favor in recent years, however, and this is the notion that the critical period for risk factors relevant to breast cancer occurs prior to the first birth of a child. With this paradigm shift, Colditz and Frazier[49] have proposed that the risk for breast cancer is set by events of early life and that our efforts in prevention should shift focus to women in their youth. They further propose that the time between menarche and first birth is the time when there is the highest rate of breast tissue aging and when breast tissue is the most vulnerable to mutagenesis.[49] Thus, they see that age at the time of exposure to risk determinants such as irradiation, alcohol consumption, and cigarette smoking is critical, with younger age being associated with the greater risk.[49] Their literature review has shown that girls who undergo irradiation of the chest at a young age have an increased risk of breast cancer, that there is a more significant impact of alcohol consumption at a younger age, and that several studies of smoking and breast cancer have demonstrated an increased risk in those who have initiated smoking at an early age.[49]

Colditz and Frazier[49] also present some new options for prevention based on this paradigm that would include (1) decreasing the period from menarche to first birth or (2) preventing the accumulation of DNA damage to the breast tissue during this period through dietary factors and delaying the adoption of smoking and alcohol drinking behaviors. A reduced interval between menarche and first birth can be best achieved by increasing physical activity among preadolescent girls, and these authors speculate that a 1-year increase in age at menarche would lead to a 9% decrease in a population-wide risk of breast cancer at age 70 years.[49] Thus, we see that even if interventions were shifted to the adolescent portion of our population, the message would be similar: consume more antioxidants and folate and increase physical exercise!

III. POPULATION GENETICS AND MARKERS FOR RISK

A. Family History

It is estimated that 85% of breast cancer occurs among women without a strong genetic predisposition. King et al.[50] estimate that screening for carriers of the *BRCA1* gene that predisposes to breast cancer will only identify 15% of women who will develop breast cancer. However, the search for the gene responsible for these 15% has been feverish and relentless in the past few years. We know that family history of breast cancer is an established risk factor for this disease and is used to identify women at higher risk. Colditz et al.[51] have analyzed the impact of the nongenetic known risk factors for breast cancer against a background of family history of the disease in order to better define the risks in this group of genetically higher risk women. Data were analyzed from the Nurses' Health Study, and the known reproductive risk factors from the Pike mathematical model[52] were prospectively examined among women with and without a family history of the disease. Among women with a family history of breast cancer, the known reproductive risk factors had associations that were different from those seen in women without a positive family history. There was little protection from a later age at menarche and no protection from nulliparity vs. nulliparity, nor was there protection with earlier age at first birth.[51] These data would seem to indicate that there may be two different biological paths for the development of breast cancer, one of which would be dependent on what genes you were born with. This idea would be consistent with the "two-hit" hypothesis of multistage carcinogenesis first proposed by Knudsen in 1971.[53]

Another epigenetic factor which may influence the genetics of breast cancer would be DNA repair proficiency. Helzlsouer et al.[54] have hypothesized that the suboptimal repair of DNA damage, such as is seen in persons with ataxia telangectasia, may be a susceptibility factor which predisposes women to breast cancer through increased sensitivity to carcinogenic damage from environmental exposures such as ionizing radiation. They went on to examine the blood of control women, those with high risk, and those with breast cancer for DNA repair proficiency. They discovered that the women at high risk had fivefold increases in unrepaired DNA damage following irradiation, indicating that these individuals may have subtle defects in DNA repair or apoptosis genes which place them at increased cancer risk.

B. BRCA1

With these ideas in hand, we will now review the history of the genetics of breast cancer. A family history of breast cancer is associated with an increased risk of the disease. This is particularly so if the family history includes a woman who had early age of onset of the disease or bilateral disease. Anderson[55] has calculated an increased risk of ninefold for first-degree relatives of breast cancer cases who are premenopausal and have bilateral cancer. Segregation analyses have provided evidence for the presence of a rare dominant breast cancer gene conferring a high risk. The inherited basis of breast and/or ovarian cancer (see Chapter 4) has now been confirmed with the localization of susceptibility genes to chromosomes 17q and 13q.[56] The majority of large multiple-case families can now be attributed to BRCA1 or BRCA2. BRCA1, located on 17q, was identified in 1990 by Hall et al.[57] and has now been cloned.[58] Current estimates of the frequency of this gene from the Breast Cancer Consortium[59] indicate that the BRCA1 gene is likely to account for approximately 5–7% of all breast cancers. BRCA2, a predominantly breast cancer gene, has now been localized to chromosome 13q by linkage analysis.[60] A third locus has also been proposed.[61] The BRCA1 gene has been cloned and found to be composed of 22 coding exons and over more than 100 kb of genomic DNA.[58] Germline mutations were initially detected in five out of eight families which demonstrated linkage to BRCA1.[58] Three specific mutations appeared to be relatively common, occurring 8, 7, and 5 times out of 38 distinct mutations found.[56] It is thought that BRCA1 acts as a tumor-suppressor gene, in that cancers in BRCA1-linked families result from the inheritance of an inactivating mutation in one copy of the gene, followed by a somatic (acquired) mutation in the nonmutant copy of the gene on the other chromosome. Breast cancers in BRCA1-linked families do occur at an earlier age than in the general population, and based on a gene frequency of 0.002 for mutant BRCA1 alleles, the proportion of breast cancers due to BRCA1 in the population is 28% in those less than 30 years and only 1% in women over 70 years.[62] The evidence thus far suggests that BRCA1 may not be critical in the development of the majority of breast and ovarian cancers.[56]

C. BRCA2

A second breast cancer susceptibility gene (BRCA2) has been reported to be localized to chromosome 13q12-13.[60] Although the tumor-suppressor gene RB1 is in the same region, it has been clarified that BRCA2 is not RB1. The evidence thus far has indicated that BRCA2 is also a tumor-suppressor gene. Like BRCA1,

BRCA2 appears to confer a high risk of early onset of breast cancer in females.[56] Studies are under way to estimate the penetrance of the *BRCA2* gene and whether or not mutations in this gene cause other cancers besides breast and ovarian. Berman et al.[63] have recently reported that there is a common mutation in *BRCA2* that predisposes to a variety of cancers found in both Jewish Ashkenazi and non-Jewish individuals. Ford and Easton[56] have concluded that "it is now clear that most breast-ovarian cancer families are caused by *BRCA1* and some, possibly all, of the remainder are due to *BRCA2*."

There are a number of families characterized by early-onset female breast cancer and/or male breast cancer which show no linkage to either *BRCA1* or *BRCA2*, and it was thought[56] that one more breast cancer gene with a high penetrance was yet to be discovered. Sobel et al.[64] have attempted to localize the putative *BRCA3* gene and as such have conducted linkage and loss of heterozygosity analyses in a panel of French families with breast tumors. Although their results have not reached significance, they support the existence of a putative *BRCA3* gene on chromosome 8p. They concluded that additional families needed to be tested to support this hypothesis.[64] They also suggest that this locus at 8p12-p22 is a tumor-suppressor gene, as are *BRCA1* and *BRCA2*.

D. Other Genes for Increased Risk

Other candidate genes for increased risk for breast cancer would include the *TP53* gene, *HRAS*, ataxia telangestasia (*AT* gene), and the genes associated with hereditary nonpolyposis colon cancer (*HNPCC*). In 1990, Malkin et al.[65] reported that germline mutations of the *p53* gene were present in five of five families studied with the Li-Fraumeni syndrome. However, available evidence suggests that germline *TP53* mutations account for a very small portion of breast cancer occurring outside of this syndrome.[56] Breast cancers associated with these mutations occur very young, and the effect of the *p53* gene is thought to be restricted to premenopausal breast cancer only.[62] *HRAS1* mutations are rare alleles that have been associated with cancer.[56] It is unclear whether these alleles are specifically associated with breast cancer, although some authors[66] have determined a relative risk of the occurrence of rare *HRAS1* alleles and breast cancer to be 1.68, thus accounting for as many as 1 in 11 breast cancers. A number of studies have shown that female relatives of *AT* patients are at increased risk of breast cancer.[56] It is estimated that *AT* could account for about 4% of breast cancers diagnosed below age 60 and that this relative risk decreases with age.[56]

In summary, most familial breast cancer appears to be linked to either or both *BRCA1* and *BRCA2*, with much smaller proportions of cancers attributed to mutations in the other genes we have mentioned. However, taken together, these high-penetrance genes are still only likely to account for probably less than 10% of all breast and ovarian cancer cases in the population. But risk estimates for *BRCA2* should be available soon. Also, genetic testing for *BRCA1* will soon become widely available. However, because of the size of this gene and the wide scattering of mutations throughout the gene, the information will be difficult to interpret.[56] However, through determination of very high-risk populations, we may eventually be able to intervene and prevent the second mutation causing loss of heterozygosity leading to cancer.

IV. DIETARY FAT

A. Obesity and Body Mass

The link between dietary fat and risk for breast cancer has been controversial for years (Table 2.1). For the purposes of our discussion, we will divide the dietary fat issue into actual dietary studies and those studies of breast cancer risk that are related to obesity and body mass index. With regard to breast cancer, body size has long been an interest of epidemiologists. Most studies examining height and weight support an association of height with increased breast cancer risk.[67] Hunter and Willet[68] have reviewed diet as well as body build in relation to breast cancer. The relation of height to breast cancer has been extensively studied[68] in a number of case-control as well as prospective studies. Most of the case-control studies report a modest positive association between attained height and risk of breast cancer. The relative risks for all of the studies with at least 500 cases is between 0.7 and 2.1 for all women, and only some of the studies divide their analyses into pre- and postmenopausal

Table 2.1   Studies of Body Mass and Dietary Fat and Breast Cancer Risk

Nutritional Endpoint	Association with Risk	Reference
Height/weight	Increased	Willett[67]
		Ziegler et al.[70]
Height	Increased	Reviewed by Hunter and Willett[68]
	Increased; prospective study	London et al.[69]
Body mass index	Increased	Reviewed by Hunter and Willett[68]
Body mass index/estradiol	Increased	Potischman et al.[71]
Fried foods, hard fat	Increased	Phillips[73]
Total fat intake	Increased	Miller et al.[74]
Beef, red meat, pork	Increased	Lubin et al.[75]
Fat intake	No association	Graham et al.[76]
Total fat intake; meta-analysis	Small increase	Howe et al.[77]
Total fat intake	Modest increase; prospective study	Kushi et al.[78]
	No association	Review by Hunter and Willett[68]
	No association; prospective study	Willett et al.[80]
Total fat intake; calories	Increased	Barrett-Connor and Friedlander[81]

women.[68] In the Nurses' Health Study,[69] a significant positive association was seen between height and breast cancer risk in postmenopausal women. Thus, there appears to be convincing evidence that attained height is modestly associated with breast cancer risk. This has also been recently examined in Asian-American women.[70] These authors report that height, recent adiposity (weight in current decade of life/height^2), and recent weight change were strong predictors of breast cancer risk, after adjustment was made for accepted breast cancer risk factors.[70] Risk doubled (relative risk 2.01) over the 7-inch range in height, and the effects were seen in premenopausal and postmenopausal women. Recent weight loss was consistently associated with reduced risk (relative risk 0.7) compared with no recent weight change.

Body mass index [weight (kg)/height (m)^2] and breast cancer risk have been examined in a number of studies. Most of the data available suggest an interaction between body mass index, breast cancer, and menopausal status.[68] In 11 out of 13 case-control studies of body mass index and breast cancer risk, a greater relative risk was seen for postmenopausal women in the highest body mass category, but this is seen in only 6 of 13 studies in premenopausal women.[68] A similar inverse association between weight at age 18 and risk of breast cancer has been observed for premenopausal but not postmenopausal breast cancer in the Nurses' Health Study.[69] The mechanism underlying these findings appears to be related to higher circulating levels of estrogens in obese postmenopausal women. Potischman et al.[71] investigated the relationship between body mass and hormonal profiles in a group of women who served as community and hospital control subjects from a study of endometrial cancer.[71] Results indicated that as the body mass index increased, total estradiol decreased in premenopausal women and increased in postmenopausal women. The authors speculate that the surprising finding in premenopausal women may have been due to sequestration of estradiol in adipose tissue, but no conclusions can be drawn. Another recent study of diet, hormones, and breast cancer risk[72] reported that African-American women appear to have higher levels of serum hormones than Caucasian women and that dietary intervention with a low-fat and high-fiber diet can result in the lowering of serum estrogens.

B. Dietary Fat Intake

Dietary fat intake and breast cancer risk have been studied constantly since the first observation was published in 1975, which implicated five categories of foods to be associated with breast cancer: fried foods, fried potatoes, hard fat used for frying, dairy products except milk, and white bread, with the relative risks ranging from 1.6 to 2.6.[73] In another early case-control study,[74] the strongest association for dietary factors and breast cancer risk was seen for total fat consumption in both premenopausal and postmenopausal women, although the relative risks were low, and there was no dose–response. Yet another study reported that the relative risk of breast cancer increased significantly with more frequent consumption of beef and other red meat, pork, and sweet desserts.[75] However, more recent studies have not supported the connection between dietary fat and breast cancer risk. Hunter and Willett[68] have extensively reviewed the literature on studies of dietary fat and breast cancer risk. The largest case-control study thus far has been that of Graham et al.,[76] who compared the fat intake of 2024 breast cancer cases with 1463 controls and found that both animal fat and total fat intake were nearly identical in the two groups. A number of other smaller case-control studies have been summarized by Howe et al.[77] in a meta-analysis which included 4312 cases and 5978 controls. When total fat intake was analyzed as a continuous variable, significant positive associations were observed in four studies, nonsignificant positive associations were seen in six, and inverse associations were seen in two. However, when all the data were pooled, a significant but weak association was observed for both total and saturated fat in postmenopausal women.[77] The pooled relative risk was 1.35 for a 100-g increase in total daily fat intake, although the risk was slightly higher for postmenopausal women (1.48). Also supporting the same hypothesis, Kushi et al.[78] reported a modest positive association of total fat intake with risk of breast cancer in a cohort study of 34,388 postmenopausal women from Iowa.

In prospective studies of dietary fat and breast cancer risk, 10 studies with at least 50 incident cases of breast cancer were analyzed by Hunter and Willett.[68] The total number of breast cancer cases in the 10 studies from 1987 through 1993 was 3580, which is similar to the number in the pooled analysis by Howe et al.[77] In not one study was a significant association observed when the highest category of intake was compared with the lowest, and the average relative risk for all ten studies was 1.03.[68] Only one study[79] had a somewhat high relative risk (1.72), and in this one, before adjustment for energy intake, the relative risk was only 0.85. In the largest prospective cohort study, the Nurses' Health Study,[80] 89,494 women were followed for 8 years, and the relative risk for developing breast cancer for the highest quintile of dietary fat intake was only 0.86, indicating no effect of this dietary factor on the risk of developing breast cancer. However, the controversy still rages, and new studies still emerge to fuel the controversy. Barrett-Connor and Freidlander[81] in a more recent prospective study reported that cases had significantly higher age-adjusted intake of fat and that women with cancer had consumed more calories, protein, and carbohydrates than did other subjects. These results support the hypothesis that total calorie consumption, as well as dietary fat consumption, is a risk factor for breast cancer in postmenopausal women.

In terms of dietary fat and breast cancer, there have been many attempts to reconcile the positive correlations from international studies with the lack of positive findings from case-control and prospective studies. Some workers in the field have proposed that dietary self-report instruments may be inadequate for the analytic epidemiologic studies of dietary fat and disease risk because of measurement error bias.[82] The author cites growing evidence that total energy and, presumably, both total fat and percent energy from fat are increasingly underreported as percent body fat increases.[82] It is hoped by many that the dietary interventions in the Women's Health Trial[83] will put some of the controversy to rest. However, those who believe the most current of the dietary fat and breast cancer hypotheses (that dietary fat reduction at an early age may reduce breast cancer risk decades later) are not so sure.[68]

V. ANTIOXIDANT VITAMINS (A, C, AND E)

A. Vitamin A and Carotenoids

In discussing the antioxidant nutrients and breast cancer, we will limit our discussion to the micronutrients vitamin A, vitamin C, and vitamin E (Table 2.2). Selenium will be discussed in a later section. Antioxidant micronutrients and breast cancer risk have been the subject of several studies, but no strong consistent relationship appears to have emerged. Vitamin A consists of both preformed vitamin A as retinol and retinyl esters, as well as the carotenoids found primarily in fruits and vegetables. A number of case-control studies have examined the role of vitamin A intake, and all have found a protective association.[67] Willett and Hunter[84] have extensively reviewed the epidemiologic evidence for vitamin A and breast, colon, and prostate cancers. A large number of studies have assessed the association between vitamin A intake and breast cancer risk.[84] Most studies have been case-control studies and have defined the relative risks associated with high vs. low intakes of either preformed vitamin A, carotenoid vitamin A, or total vitamin A. Only four of the

Table 2.2 Studies of Antioxidant Vitamins and Breast Cancer Risk

Vitamin	Association with Risk	Reference
Vitamin A intake	Inverse	Review in 67, 99
	Inverse, slight	100
	Inverse, slight; combined analysis	77
Preformed vitamin A intake	Inverse, slight	85–88
	No association	89–92
Carotenoids intake	Slight inverse; 10 of 13 studies	76, 85–97
Beta-carotene intake	Inverse	101, 110
Beta-carotene, blood	Inverse	94, 102
Beta-carotene, serum	Direct	104
Beta-carotene, adipose tissue	No association	106
Retinol, plasma	No association	94
Vitamin E	Inverse	101, 110
	No association	99
	Two of five no or direct association	67
Vitamin C	No association	76
	Inverse	97, 110
	Inverse; meta-analysis	77

case-control studies that reported on preformed vitamin A intake found slight decreases in risk with higher intake,[85-88] and another four studies found no association.[89-92] There have been to date 13 studies reporting on the risk of breast cancer associated with the dietary intake of carotenoids.[76,85-97] Ten of these have reported relative risks of 0.8 or less, with three reporting relative risks of 1.0–1.2. Howe et al.[77] conducted a combined analysis of original data from 12 studies of diet and breast cancer and found the relative risks for the highest quintile of total vitamin A intake were 0.87 for postmenopausal women and the relative risk for beta-carotene intake was 0.8. In summary, the data from all case-control studies are consistent with a slight protective effect of higher vitamin A intakes, with a stronger association for beta-carotene than for preformed vitamin A. Several prospective studies have been published in recent years.[98-100] In the Nurses' Health Study, Hunter et al.[99] prospectively studied the cohort of 89,494 women and assessed their intake of vitamins A, C, and E from foods and supplements at baseline and in 1984. They found a significant inverse association of vitamin A intake with risk of breast cancer (relative risk 0.8). In a previous study of postmenopausal women in New York, Graham et al.[100] reported that there was from highest to lowest quintiles of intake relative risks of 0.96 for total vitamin A, 0.93 for preformed vitamin A, and 0.89 for beta-carotene. The most recent case-control study of intake of selected micronutrients and breast cancer risk is from Italy.[101] Results from this study showed a significant inverse correlation between dietary intake of beta-carotene, vitamin E, and calcium and the risk of breast cancer. The major sources of beta-carotene and vitamin E were various raw vegetables, including vegetable oils used for seasoning.[101]

Data from studies of blood levels of beta-carotene and risk of breast cancer in women are less supportive than the dietary data.[86,88,94,102-104] Only one case-control study[94] and one prospective study[102] showed reduced risks for women with high beta-carotene levels. Potischman et al.[94] reported that there was no overall association between plasma retinol and breast cancer, but a positive relationship was observed between retinol and breast cancer in a subgroup with low plasma beta-carotene values, suggesting that low plasma beta-carotene may be a risk factor for breast cancer. In contrast, in a Finnish study, Knekt et al.[104] reported a substantial increase in risk among women in the highest category of serum beta-carotene level, similar to the results also in Finland from the ATBC trial in lung cancer.[105] A recent case-control study in Europe by the European Community Multicentre Study on Antioxidants, Myocardial Infarction, and Cancer of the Breast (EURAMIC) was performed on adipose tissue to determine levels of alpha-tocopherol and beta-carotene.[106] Mean antioxidant levels did not differ significantly after adjustment for age and center. Odds ratios for highest vs. lowest tertiles of exposure were 1.15 for vitamin E, 0.74 for beta-carotene, and 0.96 for selenium.[106] These results do not support the hypothesis that antioxidant nutrients are important determinants of breast cancer risk.

Two intervention studies are currently under way to study the efficacy of retinoid or carotenoid compounds to prevent occurrence of breast cancer.[107, 108] In an Italian study,[107] fenretinamide (4-HPR), a synthetic retinoid, is being used in a trial of women who already have breast cancer to determine chemopreventive efficacy against recurrence of cancer in the contralateral breast.[107] Also, in the United States, Buring and colleagues are conducting a randomized trial, known as the Women's Health Study, to determine if beta-carotene can affect risk for breast and other cancers in women.[108] Another recent study has examined the relationship between carotenoid intake, plasma lutein concentrations, and estrogen receptor status in older women diagnosed with breast cancer.[109] They found that a carotenoid-rich diet may improve prognosis after a breast cancer diagnosis.

B. Vitamin E

There have been few published studies linking vitamin E and breast cancer. The recent Italian study by Negri et al.[101] found significant inverse associations between breast cancer risk and dietary intake of vitamin E. This was a case-control study, but the largest prospective study published, the Nurses' Health Study,[99] did not show any protective effect for vitamin E. Three earlier case-control studies have reported protective associations, whereas another two report no effect or a direct effect.[67]

C. Vitamin C

Vitamin C has also been infrequently studied. In a New York State study by Graham et al.,[76] vitamin C was not found to be protective, but in a subsequent study a protective effect was seen for vitamin C.[97] Howe et al.[77] in their meta-analysis of dietary factors and breast cancer from 12 case-control studies observed a significant inverse association for ascorbic acid and breast cancer risk. The relative risk for breast cancer for highest vs. lowest quintile of intake for vitamin C was 0.69 in the study by Howe et al. These authors speculate that "if all postmenopausal women in the population were to increase fruit and vegetable intakes to reach an average daily consumption of vitamin C totaling 380 mg/day, the risk of breast cancer in the population of postmenopausal women in North America would be reduced by 16%."[77]

D. Vegetables and Fruits

A recent study focused on premenopausal breast cancer risk and intake of vegetables, fruits, and related nutrients.[110] A number of previous studies have reported data that indicated that a diet high in vegetables and fruits may protect against breast cancer.[110] However, most of these studies surveyed a number of dietary factors and did not look at the specific nutrients that may be present in the fruits and vegetables. The recent study by Freudenheim et al.[110] was a case-control study of diet, including the intake of nonfood supplements, and premenopausal breast cancer risk. They evaluated in detail the intake of vegetables, fruits, vitamins C and E, folic acid, individual carotenoids, and dietary fiber with its components. The results indicated significant reductions in risk for vitamin C (odds ratio = 0.53), alpha-tocopherol (odds ratio = 0.55), folic acid (odds ratio = 0.50), alpha-carotene (odds ratio = 0.67), beta-carotene (odds ratio = 0.46), lutein + zeaxanthin (odds ratio = 0.47), and dietary fiber from fruits and vegetables (odds ratio = 0.48). No association with risk was found for beta-cryptoxanthin, lycopene, or grain fiber. Fruits were weakly associated with a reduction in risk (odds ratio = 0.67), and no association was found between breast cancer risk and the intake of vitamins C and E and folic acid as supplements. The authors concluded that in this population of premenopausal women, the intake of vegetables appears to reduce breast cancer risk.[110]

In summary, the data on dietary intake of antioxidant nutrients appear to demonstrate a small protective effect for vitamin A and, in some cases, for vitamins E and C. However, these micronutrients may only be biochemical markers for consumption of a large amount of fruits and vegetables, which contain so much more than just the nutrients analyzed. We will discuss phytochemicals in a later section.

VI. SELENIUM

Selenium is an essential trace element that has been studied for years for its relationship to the risk for breast and other cancers (Table 2.3). A number of ecologic studies have demonstrated strong inverse associations between selenium exposure and breast cancer.[111–113] There have also been a number of studies which have examined the levels of selenium in the blood and toenails, as well as in the diet, and correlated these findings to the risk for breast cancer. Basu et al.[114] examined serum concentrations of several antioxidant nutrients, including selenium, in 89 women who had either breast cancer, benign breast

Table 2.3 Studies of Selenium Intake or Status and Breast Cancer Risk

Selenium Measure	Association with Risk	Reference
Selenium intake	Inverse	111–113
	No association	117
Serum selenium	Inverse	114, 115, 121
Serum glutathione peroxidase	Inverse	116, 121
Plasma selenium	Inverse	122
	No association; prospective study	117, 119, 120, 124
Toenail selenium	No association	117, 125

disease, or no breast pathology at all and found lower serum levels of vitamins A, E, and beta-carotene, as well as selenium. However, these authors[114] concluded that these low serum levels may be merely a consequence of the disease in general. Chaitchik et al.[115] examined the distribution of selenium in blood samples of women in Israel with breast cancer as well as healthy matched controls. They found a weighted mean value of 0.076 ppm selenium in the blood of breast cancer patients vs. 0.119 ppm selenium in the healthy controls, which was significantly lower. They concluded there was also an inverse association between stage and selenium concentration, although these were only small sample sizes.[115] In a recent case-control study in Sweden,[116] plasma selenium and glutathione peroxidase (GPX) in erythrocytes were analyzed. In individuals without supplemental selenium intake, a preventive effect for breast cancer was found, increasing with plasma selenium level. This was significant for women over 50 years of age, and a nonsignificant effect was also seen in women under 50.[116]

Dietary studies of selenium and breast cancer show mixed results. Van't Veer et al.[117] measured selenium in the diet, plasma, and toenails of breast cancer cases and controls in a Netherlands study. No statistically significant trend was observed in the odds ratios for any of the selenium indicators analyzed. These authors concluded that there was no substantial association between selenium and breast cancer risk for either short-term or long-term markers of selenium status.[117] A subsequent analysis of the dietary data in this study[118] resulted in a lowered odds ratio of 0.40 for those women who consumed a favorable dietary pattern which included a high intake of beta-carotene and selenium, but this was found to be more attributable to the low intake of fat and high intake of fermented milk products than to selenium. Gerber et al.[119] performed a case-control study of breast cancer patients in Montpelier, France, and examined the blood and cellular levels of selenium and vitamins E and C. They found that the levels of these antioxidants were overall higher in cases than controls, and the results were slightly modified when adjustment was made for exclusion of vitamin pill users. No significant findings were reported for selenium, however.[119] Another case-control study of serum selenium levels was reported from Finland.[120] Serum selenium values were 0.79 µg/l in cases and 81 µg/l in controls. The authors concluded that there was no association between selenium levels and breast cancer risk.[120] In contrast, Pawlowicz et al.[121] examined selenium concentrations in whole blood and plasma, as well as the activity of red cell and plasma GPX. Cancer patients were found to have significantly lower whole blood and plasma selenium concentrations, as well as lower GPX activities, compared to the values found for healthy controls, and these authors concluded that this may be indicative of increased cancer risk.[121] It is also a consideration that in those studies which have shown a decreased selenium level for breast cancer patients, this is a consequence of their disease. Gupta et al.[122] examined the plasma selenium level in cancer patients in India and found that there was a significantly lowered level (70 ng/ml) in breast cancer patients compared with controls (117 ng/ml). The selenium level was found to decrease with the progress of disease and recurrence of disease, thus adding credence to the idea that most case-control studies have found lowered selenium levels to merely reflect the consequences of the disease. This concept was taken one step farther by Sharma et al.,[123] who reported the use of serum levels of trace elements including selenium for diagnosis and prognosis of breast malignancies.

Hunter et al.[124] performed one of the few prospective studies of selenium status and breast cancer risk. They collected toenail clippings from 62,641 women in the Nurses' Health Study cohort at a time when they were free of cancer. During 53 months of follow-up, 434 cases of breast cancer were diagnosed among those women for whom there were toenail clippings, and these were matched to controls. The mean selenium level in toenails from cases was 0.83 µg/g, and for controls it was 0.821. The authors conclude from their data that although they cannot exclude a possible influence of selenium intake before adulthood, the selenium status later in life does not appear to be an important risk factor in the etiology of breast cancer.[124] Another more recent toenail selenium study by van den Brandt et al.[125] was performed on Dutch women in a prospective study of breast cancer cases diagnosed within 3.3 years of follow-up. They reported significantly lower selenium levels among cases diagnosed early in follow-up, but when these cases were excluded from the analysis, there was no significant trend. The authors found no evidence from their prospective data to support an association between selenium status and breast cancer.[125] A study by Garland et al.[126] assessed the reproducibility of paired specimens over a 6-year period of using toenails as a source for biomarker data. They concluded that toenail levels of certain trace elements are useful biomarkers of exposure if only one sample is assumed to represent long-term exposure, but that substantial attenuation of measures of association can occur due to random within-person variability of exposure. Thus, the reliability of this measurement should be considered when interpreting these studies of long-term trace element exposure and cancer risk.

More recently, Garland et al.[126] reviewed much of the epidemiologic evidence on the relationship between the antioxidant nutrients, including selenium, and breast cancer risk. These authors concluded that for selenium, a substantial body of evidence indicates a lack of any appreciable effect of selenium intake on breast cancer risk, at least within the range of human diets. They go on to make the recommendation that all future studies should be prospective in design, and that certain methodological issues, such as appropriate handling and storage of blood specimens, should be addressed.[126] Clark et al.[127] performed a selenium supplementation intervention trial on nonmelanoma skin cancer patients over a 7-year period. Although they reported that there was no decreased incidence of recurrence of skin cancer in the selenium-treated arm of this study, there was a significant decrease in cancer mortality, and this was specific for lung, colon, and prostate cancers, but not for breast cancer. Thus, by performing the ultimate intervention experiment, no effects of selenium supplementation (at the same nontoxic doses) were seen on the incidence of breast cancer.

VII. VITAMIN D

An inverse epidemiologic correlation between sunlight availability as a source of vitamin D and the risk of breast cancer in the United States and Canada has been reported by Garland et al.[128] These findings were also substantiated in the U.S.S.R. as well.[129] Thus, the important question of vitamin D and its association with breast cancer risk has been posed. Dietary vitamin D deficiency is considered to be a risk factor for mammary carcinogenesis in rodents.[130,131] This is hypothesized to be due to an interaction between vitamin D and calcium and their effects on lessening the induced hyperproliferation by high dietary fat.[131] There has been an interest in the connection between vitamin D and breast cancer risk, especially since the current vitamin D and calcium dietary intake in the United States is far below the RDA value in all female age groups, especially for the elderly.[131] However, there is only one reported study investigating the hypothesis that vitamin D deficiency is etiological in the development of cancer of the breast,[132] and this study demonstrated no differences between cases and controls in their mean daily intake of vitamin D. These authors found in a Montreal case-control study[132] that the mean daily intake of vitamin D of breast cancer cases was 1.65 IU/kg, while in the controls matched for age, the mean intake was 1.34 IU/kg. The authors pointed out that in the 5 years prior to diagnosis, the cancer patients had not increased significantly their consumption of foods rich in vitamin D, and the data also showed that twice as many cases as controls had a higher consumption of vitamin D. Thus, it does not appear that vitamin D plays a significant role in human breast cancer.

Experimentally, however, the vitamin in its active form has demonstrated protective effects in inhibiting the growth of breast cancer cells in culture[133–135] and also against the growth of tumors induced chemically in rodents.[136] In terms of human breast cancer, a curious finding is that patients with vitamin D receptor–positive tumors had a longer disease-free survival than those with receptor-negative tumors[137] and that the presence of vitamin D receptors on tumors may have potential as a prognostic indicator.[137] However, the control of cell proliferation by vitamin D compounds appears to be a separate phenomenon from the dietary and/or sunlight-derived vitamin D influences and has been reviewed previously by Pence and Dunn.[136] Therefore, it appears at this time that the data do not support a role for vitamin D functioning as a nutrient in the etiology of human breast cancer.

Table 2.4   Studies of Alcohol Consumption and Breast Cancer Risk

Type of Study	Association with Risk	Reference
Case-control	Direct	142, 143, 150, 151
	Inverse	144
Case-control, combined analysis	Direct; relative risks >1.69	139, 140
	Direct; 38 studies	141
Meta-analysis	Direct; strong dose–response	138

VIII. ALCOHOL CONSUMPTION

There have been a number of published reviews (Table 2.4) of the association between alcoholic beverage consumption and the risk for breast cancer.[138–141] The interest in this link between alcohol and breast cancer was first reported by Williams and Horm[142] in 1977, in a case-control analysis of many cancer sites in relation to alcohol consumption and cigarette smoking. This finding apparently received little attention until 1982 when Rosenberg et al.[143] reported an association between alcohol and breast cancer, which was maintained whether cancer or noncancer controls were used and also after allowance for many of the established risk factors for the disease. This publication appeared to provoke many other investigators to examine this association and also to perform meta-analyses of these accumulated studies.

The first of these reviews analyzed the association between alcohol and breast cancer risk in a combined analysis of six dietary case-control studies.[139] These six studies were from Argentina, Australia, Canada, Greece, and two from Italy, involving 1575 cases and 1974 controls. The basic unit of alcohol exposure was in grams of ethanol per day, and consumption was defined as either beer, wine, or spirits. There was also available for each study dietary data in terms of estimated daily intake from full diet histories. The results of this review of six studies are that for consumption under 40 g/day, there is an overall lack of association, and the relative risk for all drinkers of alcohol compared to nondrinkers is 1.0.[139] However, for women who consume 40 g or more alcohol per day (four drinks of spirits, three to four glasses of wine, or three to four beers per day), there is a statistically significant elevated risk for breast cancer compared with nondrinkers (relative risk = 1.69). Furthermore, the data were essentially unchanged by adjustment for the classic nondietary risk factors for breast cancer. An analysis of the relative risks by type of alcoholic beverage indicated that the effects seen are due to alcohol itself rather than any particular alcohol-containing beverage.[139]

Rosenberg et al. in 1993[140] also reviewed the epidemiologic evidence linking alcohol consumption and risk of breast cancer in 18 case-control studies in the United States and other countries. With the exception of one study[144] which suggested an inverse association between alcohol consumption and breast cancer risk and four[145–148] which had risk estimates less than 1.2, the remainder of the studies reviewed demonstrated some positive associations with relative risk estimates of 1.8 or above.[140] The strongest positive associations were observed in hospital-based studies which were conducted in France or Italy, whereas those studies which used population-based controls showed weaker associations. However, there were many inconsistencies in the studies which showed positive associations, such as the level of consumption, a lack of consistent dose–response effect, and the type of alcoholic beverage implicated in the increased risk. However, the authors conclude that the associations between alcoholic beverage consumption and breast cancer have been weak and inconsistent and that confounding cannot be ruled out. The proposed biologic mechanisms for the associations seen are speculative and poorly understood.

Another review of published case-control studies of alcoholic beverages and breast cancer by Roth et al.[141] identified 38 case-control studies which investigated possible associations between alcoholic beverages and cancer of the female breast. The major findings of these authors were similar to that of Rosenberg et al.[140] in that there was a striking difference between hospital- and community-based control studies. They further analyzed these differences by the characteristics of their study design and found that a significant association between alcohol consumption was rarely reported in studies using community-based controls[141] and that there was also no dose–response relationship in these same types of studies. The authors conclude that their findings of much lower odds ratios and dose–response slopes in those studies using population-based controls cast significant doubt on the hypothesis linking alcohol causally to human breast cancer.

A recent review study by Longnecker[138] is a meta-analysis of 38 epidemiologic studies on female breast cancer risk and alcohol consumption. This study was a follow-up to a study previously published by Longnecker et al.[149] which had reportedly found strong evidence of a dose–response association but lack of evidence of causality. The more recent study evaluated the new accumulated data and searched for unknown factors which might explain the data differences. The analysis by Longnecker et al. demonstrated a strong dose–response relationship, but the slope of the dose–response curve was very modest.[138] Interestingly, those countries with the highest per capita alcohol consumption had the strongest associations, which may reflect drinking starting at younger ages. The author also found that those studies with the longest follow-up period had weaker associations. His assessment of whether alcohol consumption causes breast cancer considers that the evidence is inconclusive at this time.

Since the 1994 meta-analysis was published, several new case-control studies have been reported. Two of these have shown positive relationships. One is a study from Spain which showed a dose–response relationship in that even at moderate levels of alcohol intake (less than 8 g/day), there was a 50% increase in risk of breast cancer, and consumption over 20 g/day was associated with a 70% elevation in risk.[150] Another study from Greece indicated a threshold effect.[151] A population-based case-control study in Sweden showed a clear increase in risk for the highest quartile of alcohol intake vs. the lowest,[152] but the effects were null when alcohol consumption was treated as a continuous variable in the analysis. In contrast, in the United Kingdom, a case-control study in young women showed no alcohol-related risk.[153]

Some plausible biologic mechanisms for the association between alcohol and breast cancer involve the effects on circulating levels of estrogenic hormones. Reichman et al.[154] have reported that in a controlled diet study, alcohol consumption was associated with statistically significant increases in levels of several estrogenic hormones and that this could be a possible explanation for the positive association seen between alcohol consumption and breast cancer. Dorgan et al.[155] have followed up on that by measuring plasma levels of estrone, estrone sulfate, estradiol, androstenedione, and dehydroepiandosterone sulfate and found that alcohol was significantly positively associated with the average level of plasma androstenedione in premenopausal women. These authors concluded that the increased risk of breast cancer related to alcohol ingestion does not appear to be mediated by elevated plasma estrogen levels. So the issue of the biologic causality for alcohol consumption is also inconsistent, and further research is warranted.

IX. PHYTOESTROGENS

Phytoestrogens are another dietary component that may be associated with a protective effect against breast cancer risk. It has been suggested that dietary phytoestrogens, which are present in legumes and grains, provide potential prevention of estrogen-dependent cancers such as breast cancer. Most of the data so far have come from cell culture and animal studies, and few human studies have been reported.[156] However, a recent study by Adlercreutz et al.[157] demonstrated that these compounds in the diet (lignans, plant heterocyclic phenols similar in structure to estrogens, and isoflavonoids) may affect the uptake and metabolism of sex hormones in postmenopausal women and thus may inhibit cancer cell growth by competing for estrogen binding sites.

A. Soy

Soy foods appear to have an important role in the prevention of cancer.[158] Several phytochemical components of soy have been reported to have a role in cancer prevention, especially breast cancer. Most of the studies with soy derivatives have centered on genistein. Most of these studies have been in cell culture or animal models. However, there have been several epidemiologic studies showing that a high intake of soy foods is associated with a reduced risk of breast cancer.[159, 160] It has also been used as one explanation for the differences seen in breast cancer incidence between Asian and American women, because Asians consume a diet rich in soy products. Wu et al.[160] recently conducted a population-based case-control study of breast cancer among Asian women, and their analysis compared the usual adult intake of soy (estimated primarily from tofu intake) among breast cancer cases and control women. The risk of breast cancer decreased with increasing frequency of intake of tofu after adjustment for age, study area, ethnicity, and migration history. The protective effect of a high tofu intake was observed in pre- and postmenopausal women. However, the authors did caution that they cannot discount the possibility that soy intake is a marker of other protective aspects of the Asian diet and/or Asian lifestyle.[160]

B. Flaxseed

Mammalian lignans, which are produced in the colon from precursors in foods, have been suggested as playing a role in the cancer-protective effect of vegetarian diets.[156, 161] Flaxseed meal and flaxseed flour have been shown to produce the greatest amount of these protective lignans following colonic bacterial fermentation[161] and as such have been promoted in recent years as a cancer-protective source of dietary fiber.[156] Although the evidence that lignans can reduce the risk of human cancer is still unclear, many have been shown to have antitumor, antimitotic, antioxidant, and antiestrogenic properties.[161] Recently, flaxseed ingestion has been shown to modulate the menstrual cycle, with possible relevance to reducing breast cancer risk.[162]

X. PHYTOCHEMICALS

A plant-derived dietary factor which has received a lot of attention in recent years for its association with reduction in risk for a number of cancers is green and black tea. Since tea is one of the most frequently consumed beverages in the world, there have been a number of cell and animal model studies on the anticarcinogenic properties of both green and black tea. Black tea is thought to be less anticarcinogenic than green tea, because most of the catechin compounds have been oxidized to forms that are less active. Goldbohm et al.[163] have recently published a cohort study in which they examined black tea consumption and the subsequent risks of a number of cancers, including breast. The results indicate that the relative risk of breast cancer among consumers of five or more cups of tea per day was 1.3, and no dose–response association was seen.[163] Similar lack of association was seen for other major cancers, and the authors concluded that their study does not support the hypothesis that consumption of black tea protects against four of the major human cancers. However, there was no enhancing effect seen either.[163]

XI. COOKED MEAT MUTAGENS

The significance of red meat as a risk factor for human breast cancer has been considered since 1981. However, the connection between the consumption of red meat has been more prominently linked to the development of colon cancer until quite recently. To review the literature involving meat and colon cancer, see Chapter 6 in this volume. The first reports of an increased risk for breast cancer with more frequent consumption of beef and other red meat were in 1981, and only a slight increase in relative risk was reported.[164] This was rapidly followed by three other reports that showed either no protection in a nonmeat-eating group of nuns compared with those who did eat meat[165] or no association of breast cancer with meat intake.[166, 167] Another negative finding in Seventh-Day Adventist females did not demonstrate any association with frequency of consumption of meat.[168] However, beginning in the 1990s, a number of studies were emerging linking red meat consumption with breast cancer. Van den Brandt et al.[169] reported that in a Netherlands population, the odds ratio for eating meat rarely vs. regularly was 1.75. Vatten et al.[170] reported that in a Norwegian population, the RR for eating meat more than five times per week was 1.8. This was also found to be the case in a Singapore population.[96] By the mid-1990s, there were more studies reporting an increased risk for breast cancer for eating meat, and this was seen in a number of populations. Toniolo et al.[171] found in New York women a relative risk of 1.87 with increased consumption of meat. Landa et al.[172] reported the highest relative risk of 3.20 for processed meat intake in Spain, as did Gaard et al.[173] in Norway, who reported a relative risk of 2.44 for eating meat more than five times a week. There were also several reports of negative associations. Matos et al.[174] found in Argentina only an insignificant trend, and Boyd et al.[175] found the relative risk for meat consumption was only 1.18. In summary, in the most recent and most compelling report from Uruguay,[176] with a relative risk of 4.2 for increased consumption of well-cooked meat notwithstanding, of a total of 15 epidemiological reports in the literature, only 8 demonstrated an increased risk with eating meat for breast cancer, and 7 showed either a null or a weak association.

The experimental studies do not solve the dilemma either. The only experimental studies reported to date are concerned with the abilities of the heterocyclic amines (HCAs), food-derived mutagens, to induce mammary cancer in rodents. There are only three of these studies, and they have used extremely high amounts of these HCAs to elicit the development of mammary cancer in rodents. In long-term feeding studies with rats, the HCA PhIP has been shown to cause carcinomas in the mammary gland and colon.[177] However, the compound PhIP was given in the diet at 400 ppm for 52 weeks and resulted in a tumor incidence of 47% in F344 rats. Two additional HCAs, IQ and MeIQ, have also been shown to cause mammary gland cancer in rodents. Kato et al.[178] fed MeIQ to F344 rats at 0.03% of the diet for 40 weeks and induced mammary tumors in 25% of the rats. Tanaka et al.[179] had also fed multiple doses of IQ to Sprague-Dawley rats for 31 weeks and induced mammary tumors in 44% of the rats. However, since PhIP is quantitatively the most prevalent of these three HCA carcinogens in cooked meats that are staples of the Western diet, it is most probably PhIP that is the etiologic agent in human breast cancer.[180]

XII. CAFFEINE

The idea that caffeine might be involved in the etiology of breast disease was first proposed in 1979.[181] Since that time, numerous experimental and epidemiologic studies have evaluated the relationship between methylxanthines and breast disease (reviewed by Lubin and Ron[181]). All previous studies except one have concluded that caffeine does not play a role in the development of breast cancer, although there have been suggestions that caffeine exacerbates fibrocystic disease.[182] In the Iowa Women's Health Study, caffeine intake was assessed by a food frequency questionnaire, and there was no apparent association between breast cancer occurrence and quintile of caffeine intake, even after adjustment for multiple breast cancer risk factors.[183] Therefore, we can conclude at this time that no recommendations are necessary concerning caffeine consumption.

XIII. PESTICIDES

Increased attention has focused in recent years on environmental exposures that may elevate the risk of human breast cancer. Recent attention has been drawn to the issue of organochlorine residues and breast cancer. This has been the subject of a recent review.[184] A pilot study has been undertaken to measure and compare the levels of chemical residues in mammary adipose tissue from women with malignant and nonmalignant breast disease.[185] Elevated levels of polychlorinated biphenyls (PCBs), bis(4-chlorophenyl)-1,1-dichloroethane (DDE), and bis(4-chlorophenyl)-1,1,1-trichloroethane (DDT) were reported in the fat samples from women with breast cancer compared to those samples from women with benign breast disease. Although these results are just preliminary, the data suggest that there may be a role for pesticides in the etiology of human breast cancer. Wolff et al.[186] performed a blinded study to determine whether exposure to PCBs and DDE, the major metabolite of DDT, was associated with breast cancer risk in women. They analyzed sera from 14,290 participants enrolled in the New York University Women's Health Study. Their results show that the mean levels of DDE and PCBs were higher for breast cancer cases than controls, but paired differences were significant only for DDE. After adjustment for classic breast cancer risk factors such as family history and age at first pregnancy, they reported a fourfold increase in relative

risk of breast cancer for an elevation of serum DDE concentration from 2.0 ng/
ml to 191 ng/ml. There was not a significant association with PCBs. The
authors state that environmental chemical contamination may be an important
etiologic factor in breast cancer.[186] These findings suggest that considering the
widespread dissemination of these agents in the food chain, there are implications that this could be a dietary etiological agent for human breast cancer.

XIV. GENERAL CONCLUSIONS, SUMMARY, AND IMPLICATIONS

Breast cancer risk factors have been studied more extensively than those for
any other cancer that occurs in women. In general, reproductive factors such as
age at menarche, age at menopause, pregnancy, lactation, and menstrual cycle
length seem to be major determinants of breast cancer probability. In addition,
family history has also been a strong predictor of risk, especially with those
women carrying germline mutations in the BRCA genes for susceptibility.
Although the genetic link predominates in only about 10% of breast cancers,
there is still much we need to know about the function of the BRCA genes and
their interaction with environmental factors such as cigarette smoking, HRT
use, and dietary practices. For the vast majority of women diagnosed with
breast cancer, the etiology of their cancer remains completely unknown.

Obviously, breast cancer is a hormonally related cancer, and most of the
risk factors are mechanistically interpreted through that filter. However, the
data on use of oral contraceptives and HRT do not support a prominent role for
exogenous hormones in the etiology of breast cancer, although longer term
studies are needed in the case of HRT.

The general conclusions about physical exercise appear to support the idea
that increased activity tends to decrease risk. The mechanisms underlying this
observation need to be further examined. The issue of cigarette smoking and
breast cancer is still inconclusive, with the habit neither substantially decreasing nor increasing risk. However, if one chooses to agree with the Colditz and
Frazier[49] model for early intervention to reduce lifetime breast cancer risk, then
these two habits emerge as more critical determinants of risk. The messages
"more exercise" and "don't smoke" then become targeted to adolescent girls
rather than postmenopausal women. The adolescent intervention model is intriguing, and more research is needed to validate these ideas.

The controversial link between dietary fat and breast cancer risk has been
debated by the best researchers in the diet and cancer field, with no hard
conclusions to be drawn. Increased height and weight appear to modestly increase breast cancer risk, as does an increased body mass index, and these
variables are presumed to be mechanistically related to higher levels of circulating estrogens in obese postmenopausal women. Hunter and Willett[187] have

recently reviewed the epidemiologic literature on nutrition and breast cancer and have concluded that dietary fat intake in mid-life is not supportive of an association with breast cancer risk. They further state that if fat intake is relevant to breast cancer, then a relationship occurs only at low-fat intakes or during early life and recommend that future studies focus on nutrition during early life and subsequent risk of breast cancer.[187] Therefore, a strong compelling association for dietary fat is elusive, possibly due to an overlap of variables such as total calories consumed, red meat intake and its cooking preferences (i.e., generation of HCAs), body mass, and percentage body fat, all of which can be hindered by dietary assessment error bias. Finally, since the underlying cause of breast cancer appears to be related in part to estrogenic exposure, then the relationship between hormone status, dietary fat, and associated body mass variables should be more precisely assessed within the same study population. More research is also required into the dietary fat/body mass effects on estrogen metabolism across the life span of the female.

Consumption of the antioxidant vitamins A, E, and C, as well as fruits and vegetables in general, appears to be protective against breast cancer. However, we do not know if there is some property inherent in these specific vitamins which decreases risk or if increased intake is merely a marker for a healthier lifestyle. This concept of the "healthy lifestyle" may be hallmarked by a greater propensity for eating fruits and vegetables and, conversely, lower consumption of dietary fat and meat products and needs further validation. Selenium intake does not appear to modify breast cancer risk, nor does consumption of vitamin D, although both of these nutrients appear to have profound effects at pharmacologic doses in experimental animal studies.

Alcoholic beverage consumption appears to impart a modest increase in risk, although many inconsistencies exist in the data. However, the risk increase may or may not be associated with an increase in estrogenic hormones, and further research in this area is warranted.

The case for phytoestrogens, including soy isoflavones and lignans from flax, is provocative but incomplete. Most work to date has been performed in cell culture or animal models of breast cancer. More extensive data on soy in the diet of Asian women with and without breast cancer would be helpful to sort out whether a specific effect of soy or soy intake is itself a marker for the lower risk Asian lifestyle.

We still do not know the etiology of human breast cancer beyond that which appears to directly result from *BRCA1* and *BRCA2* mutations. It is possible that two mutagens contained in our foods, HCAs and pesticides, may be involved in the causation of breast cancer. The effects of these potential carcinogens need to be better assessed in future studies, both epidemiological and experimental.

Finally, in light of the fact that the strongest predictor of breast cancer risk still appears to be a family history of the disease, we need to focus future studies of other risk factors, including dietary, on the interaction of environmental risk factors with the hereditary predisposition. Dietary fat may only be a risk determinant in specific high-risk populations, and the protection afforded by fruit and vegetable consumption may also only be effective in the absence of a genetically determined risk. In a future where many women will be tested to identify their risk for breast and other cancers, perhaps studying nutritional factors by risk stratification will yield better clues as to the real role of diet in breast cancer.

REFERENCES

1. Parker, S.L., Tong, T., Bolden, S., and Wingo, P.A., Cancer statistics 1997, *CA Cancer J. Clin.*, 47, 5, 1997.
2. Whelan, S.L., Parkin, D.M., and Masuyer, E., *Patterns of Cancer in Nine Continents*, IARC Scientific Publications No. 102, International Agency for Research on Cancer, Lyon, 1990.
3. The World Health Organization Histologic Typing of Breast Tumors, 2nd ed., *Am. J. Clin. Pathol.*, 78, 1982.
4. Fisher, E.R., Gregorio, R.M., and Fisher, B., The pathology of invasive breast cancer, *Cancer*, 36, 1, 1975.
5. Rapin, V., Contesso, G., Mouriesse, H., Bertin, F., Lacombe, J.D., Piekarski, J.D., Travagli, J.P., Gadenne, C., and Friedman, S., Medullary breast carcinoma: a reevaluation of 95 cases of breast cancer with inflammatory stroma, *Cancer*, 61, 2503, 1988.
6. Rosen, P.P., Lobular carcinoma *in situ* of the breast, *Am. J. Surg. Pathol.*, 2, 225, 1978.
7. Cotran, R.S., Kumar, V., and Robbins, S.L., *Robbins Pathologic Basis of Disease*, 5th ed., W.B. Saunders, Philadelphia, 1994, chap. 24.
8. Gail, M.H., Brinton, L.A., Byar, D.P., Corle, D.K., Green, S.B., Shainer, C., and Mulvihill, J.J., Projecting individualized probabilities of developing breast cancer for white females who are being examined annually, *J. Natl. Cancer Inst.*, 81, 1879, 1989.
9. Henderson, B.E., Pike, M.C., Bernstein, L., and Ross, R.K., Breast cancer, in *Cancer Epidemiology and Prevention*, 2nd ed., Schottenfeld, D. and Fraumeni, J.F., Jr., Eds., Oxford University Press, New York, 1996, 1022.
10. Henderson, B.E., Pike, M.C., and Casagrande, J.T., Breast cancer and the oestrogen window hypothesis (letter), *Lancet*, ii, 363, 1981.
11. Henderson, B.E., Ross, R.K., Judd, H.L., Krailo, M.D., and Pike, M.C., Do regular ovulatory cycles increase breast cancer risk? *Cancer*, 56, 1206, 1985.
12. Henderson, B.E., Gerkins, V.R., Rosario, I., Casagrande, J., and Pike, M.C., Elevated serum levels of estrogen and prolactin in daughters of patients with breast cancer, *New Engl. J. Med.*, 293, 790, 1975.
13. Tanner, J., *Growth at Adolescence*, Blackwell Scientific Publishers, Oxford, 1962.
14. Feinleib, M., Breast cancer and artificial menopause: a cohort study, *J. Natl. Cancer Inst.*, 41, 315, 1968.

15. McMahon, B., Cole, P., Lin, C.R., Mirra, A.P., Ravnihar, B., Salber, E.J., Valaoras, V.G., and Yuasa, S., Age at first birth and cancer of the breast: a summary of an international study, *Bull. WHO*, 43, 209, 1970.
16. Yu, M.C., Gerkins, V.R., Henderson, B.E., Brown, J.B., and Pike, M.C., Elevated levels of prolactin in nulliparous women, *Br. J. Cancer*, 43, 826, 1981.
17. Ross, R. and Yu, M., Breast feeding and breast cancer (letter to the editor), *New Engl. J. Med.*, 330, 1683, 1994.
18. Olsson, H., Landin-Olsson, M., and Gullberg, B., Retrospective assessment of menstrual cycle length in patients with breast cancer, in patients with benign breast disease, and in women without breast disease, *J. Natl. Cancer Inst.*, 70, 17, 1983.
19. La Vecchia, C., Decarli, A., di Pietro, S., Franceschi, S., Negri, E., and Parazzini, F., Menstrual cycle patterns and the risk of breast cancer, *Eur. J. Cancer Clin. Oncol.*, 21, 417, 1985.
20. Matsumoto, S. and Nogami, Y., Statistical studies of menstruation: criticism of the definition of normal menstruation, *Gunma J. Med. Sci.*, 11, 294, 1962.
21. Kodlin, D., Winger, E.E., Morgenstern, N.L., and Chen, U., Chronic mastopathy and breast cancer, *Cancer*, 39, 2603, 1977.
22. Black, M.M., Barclay, T.H.C., Cutler, S.J., Hankey, B.F., and Asire, A.J., Association of atypical characteristics of benign breast lesions with subsequent risk of breast cancer, *Cancer*, 29, 338, 1972.
23. Dupont, W.D. and Page, D.L., Risk factors for breast cancer in women with proliferative breast disease, *New Engl. J. Med.*, 312, 146, 1985.
24. London, S.L., Connolly, J.L., Schnitt, S.J., and Colditz, G.A., A prospective study of benign breast disease and the risk of breast cancer, *J. Am. Med. Assoc.*, 267, 941, 1992.
25. Ma, L. and Boyd, N.F., Atypical hyperplasia and breast cancer risk: a critique, *Cancer Causes Control*, 3, 517, 1992.
26. Hawley, W., Nuovo, J., DeNeef, C.P., and Carter, P., Do oral contraceptive agents affect the risk of breast cancer? A meta-analysis of the case-control reports, *J. Am. Board Fam. Pract.*, 6, 123, 1993.
27. Hulka, B.S., Links between hormone replacement therapy and neoplasia, *Fertil. Steril.*, 62 (Suppl. 2), 168S, 1994.
28. Hunt, K., Vessey, M., McPherson, K., and Coleman, M., Long-term surveillance of mortality and cancer incidence in women receiving hormone replacement therapy, *Br. J. Obstet. Gynecol.*, 94, 620, 1987.
29. D'Avanzo, B., Nanni, O., La Vecchia, C., Franceschi, S., Negri, E., Giacosa, A., Conti, E., Montello, M., Talamini, R., and Decarli, A., Physical activity and breast cancer risk, *Cancer Epidemiol. Biomarkers Prev.*, 5, 155, 1996.
30. Frisch, R.E., Wyshak, G., Albright, N.L., Albright, T.E., Schiff, I., Johns, K.P., Witski, J., Shiang, E., Koff, E., and Marguglio, M., Lower prevalence of breast cancer and cancers of the reproductive system among former college athletes compared to non-athletes, *Br. J. Cancer*, 52, 885, 2985.
31. Vihko, V.J., Apter, D.L., Pukkala, E.L., Oinonen, M.T., Hakulinen, T.R., and Vihko, R.K., Risk of breast cancer among female teachers of physical education and languages, *Acta Oncol.*, 31, 201, 1992.
32. Pukkala, E., Poskiparta, M., Apter, D., and Vihko, V., Life-long physical activity and cancer risk among Finnish female teachers, *Eur. J. Cancer Prev.*, 2, 369, 1993.

33. Zheng, W., Shu, X.O., McLaughlin, J.K., Chow, W.H., Gao, Y.T., and Blot, W.J., Occupational physical activity and the incidence of cancer of the breast, corpus uteri, and ovary in Shanghai, *Cancer*, 71, 3620, 1993.

34. Dosemeci, M., Hayes, R.B., Vetter, R., Hoover, R.N., Tacker, M., Engin, K., Unsal, M., and Blair, A., Occupational physical activity, socioeconomic status, and risks of 15 cancer sites in Turkey, *Cancer Causes Control*, 4, 313, 1993.

35. Bernstein, L., Henderson, B.E., Hanisch, R., Sullivan-Halley, J., and Ross, R.K., Physical exercise and reduced risk of breast cancer in young women, *J. Natl. Cancer Inst.*, 86, 1403, 1994.

36. MacMahon, B., Trichopoulos, D., Cole, P., and Brown, J., Cigarette smoking and urinary estrogens, *New Engl. J. Med.*, 307, 1062, 1982.

37. Baron, J.A., Smoking and estrogen-related disease, *Am. J. Epidemiol.*, 119, 9, 1984.

38. Hiatt, R.A. and Fireman, B.H., Smoking, menopause, and breast cancer, *J. Natl. Cancer Inst.*, 76, 833, 1986.

39. Palmer, J.R. and Rosenberg, L., Cigarette smoking and the risk of breast cancer, *Epidemiol. Rev.*, 15, 145, 1993.

40. Sandler, D.P., Everson, R.B., and Wilcox, A.J., Cigarette smoking and breast cancer (letter), *Am. J. Epidemiol.*, 123, 370, 1986.

41. Hirayama, T., Cigarette smoking in nonsmoking women with smoking husbands based on large-scale cohort study in Japan, *Prev. Med.*, 13, 680, 1984.

42. Episteme, S., Stress and breast cancer, *Cancer J.*, 5, 129, 1992.

43. Barraclough, J., Pindor, P., Cruddas, M., Osmond, C., Taylor, I., and Perry, M., Life events and breast cancer progression, *Br. Med. J.*, 304, 1078, 1992.

44. Spiegel, D., Bloom, J.R., Kraemer, H.C., and Gottheil, E., Effect of psychosocial treatment on survival of patients with metastatic breast cancer, *Lancet*, ii, 888, 1989.

45. Longnecker, M.P., Bernstein, L., Paganini-Hill, A., Enger, S.M., and Ross, R.K., Risk factors for *in situ* breast cancer, *Cancer Epidemiol. Biomarkers Prev.*, 5, 961, 1996.

46. Pike, M.C., Henderson, B.E., Casagrande, J.T., Rosario, I., and Gray, G.E., Oral contraceptive use and early abortion as risk factors for breast cancer in young women, *Br. J. Cancer*, 43, 72, 1981.

47. Daling, J.R., Malone, K.E., Voight, L.F., White, E., and Weiss, N.S., Risk of breast cancer among young women: relationship to induced abortion, *J. Natl. Cancer Inst.*, 86, 1584, 1994.

48. Rookus, M.A. and van Leeuwen, F.E., Induced abortion and risk for breast cancer: reporting (recall) bias in a Dutch case-control study, *J. Natl. Cancer Inst.*, 88, 1759, 1996.

49. Colditz, G.A. and Frazier, A.L., Models of breast cancer show that risk is set by events of early life: prevention efforts must shift focus, *Cancer Epidemiol. Biomarkers Prev.*, 4, 567, 1995.

50. King, M., Rowell, S., and Love, S., Inherited breast and ovarian cancer. What are the risks? What are the choices? *J. Am. Med. Assoc.*, 269, 1975, 1993.

51. Colditz, G.A., Rosner, B.A., and Speizer, F.E., Risk factors for breast cancer according to family history of breast cancer, *J. Natl. Cancer Inst.*, 88, 365, 1996.

52. Pike, M.C., Krailo, M., Henderson, B., Casagrande, J., and Hoel, D., "Hormonal" risk factors, "breast tissue age" and the age-incidence of breast cancer, *Nature*, 303, 767, 1983.

53. Knudsen, A., Mutation and cancer: statistical study of retinoblastoma, *Proc. Natl. Acad. Sci. USA*, 68, 820, 1971.

54. Helzlsouer, K.J., Harris, E.L., Parshad, R., Perry, H.R., Price, F.M., and Sanford, K.K., DNA repair proficiency: potential susceptibility factor for breast cancer, *J. Natl. Cancer Inst.*, 88, 754, 1996.

55. Anderson, D.E., Genetic study of breast cancer: identification of a high-risk group, *Cancer*, 34, 1090, 1974.

56. Ford, D. and Easton, D.F., The genetics of breast and ovarian cancer, *Br. J. Cancer*, 72, 805, 1995.

57. Hall, J.M., Lee, M.K., Newman, B., Morrow, J.E., Anderson, L.A., Huey, B., and King, M.-C., Linkage of early onset familial breast cancer to chromosome 17q21, *Science*, 250, 1684, 1990.

58. Miki, Y., Swensen, J., Shattuck-Eidens, D., Futreal, P.A., Harshman, K., Tavtigian, S., Liu, Q.Y., Cochran, C., Bennett, L.M., Ding, W., Bell, R., Rosenthal, J., Hussey, C., Tran, T., McClure, M., Frye, C., Hattier, T., Phelps, R., Haugenstrano, A., Katcher, H., Yakumo, K., Gholami, Z., Shaffer, D., Stone, S., Bayer, S., Wray, C., Bogden, R., Dayananth, P., Ward, J., Tonin, P., Narod, S., Bristow, P.K., Norris, F.H., Helvering, L., Morrison, P., Rosteck, P., Lai, M., Barrett, J.C., Lewis, C., Neuhausen, S., Cannon-Albright, L., Goldgar, D., Wiseman, R., Kamb, A., and Skolnick, M.H., Isolation of *BRCA1*, the 17q-linked breast and ovarian cancer susceptibility gene, *Science*, 266, 66, 1994.

59. Easton, D.F., Bishop, D.T., Ford, D., and Crockford, G.P., The Breast Cancer Linkage Consortium, Genetic linkage analysis in familial breast and ovarian cancer: results from 214 families, *Am. J. Human Genet.*, 52, 678, 1993.

60. Wooster, R., Neuhausen, S., Manigion, J., Quirk, Y., Ford, D., Collins, N., Nguyen, K., Seal, S., Tran, T., Averill, D., Fields, P., Marshall, G., Narod, S., Lenoir, G.M., Lynch, H.T., Feunteun, J., Devilee, P., Cornelisse, C.J., Menko, F.H., Daly, P.A., Ormiston, W., McManus, R., Pye, C., Lewis, C.M., Cannon-Albright, L.A., Peto, J., Ponder, B.A.J., Skolnick, M.H., Easton, D.F., Goldgar, D.E., and Stratton, M.R., Localization of a breast cancer susceptibility gene (*BRCA2*) to chromosome 13q by genetic linkage analysis, *Science*, 265, 2088, 1994.

61. Cornelis, R.S., Cornelisse, C.J., and Devilee, P., Selection of families for predictive testing for breast cancer (letter), *Lancet*, 344, 1151, 1994.

62. Narod, S.A., Genetics of breast and ovarian cancer, *Br. Med. Bull.*, 50, 656, 1994.

63. Berman, D.B., Costalas, J., Schultz, D.C., Grana, G., Daly, M., and Godwin, A.K., A common mutation in *BRCA2* that predisposes to a variety of cancers is found in both Jewish Ashkenazi and non-Jewish individuals, *Cancer Res.*, 56, 3409, 1996.

64. Sobel, H., Kerangueven, F., Eisinger, F., Essioux, L., Noguchi, T., Gesta, P., Jacquemeier, J., Pebusque, M.-J., Bonaiti-Pellie, C., and Birnbaum, D., Indication for a possible third breast cancer predisposing gene, *BRCA3*, in the chromosome 8p12-p22 region, in *Hereditary Cancer*, Muller H., Scott, R.J., and Weber, W., Eds., Karger, Basel, 1996, 19.

65. Malkin, D., Li, F.P., Strong, L.C., Fraumeni, J.F., Nelson, C.E., Kim, D.H., Kassel, J., Gryka, M.A., Bischoff, F.Z., Tainsky, M.A., and Friend, S.H., Germline *p53* mutations in a familial syndrome of breast cancer, sarcomas and other neoplasms, *Science*, 250, 1233, 1990.
66. Krontiris, T.G., Devlin, B., Karp, D.D., Robert, N.J., and Risch, N., An association between the risk of cancer and mutations in the *HRAS1* minisatellite locus, *New Engl. J. Med.*, 329, 517, 1993.
67. Willett, W., Diet and breast cancer, *Contemp. Nutr.*, 18, 1, 1993.
68. Hunter, D.J. and Willett, W.C., Diet, body size, and breast cancer, *Epidemiol. Rev.*, 15, 110, 1993.
69. London, S.J., Colditz, G.A., Stampfer, M.J., Willett, W.C., Rossner, B., and Speizer, F.E., Prospective study of relative weight and breast cancer, *J. Am. Med. Assoc.*, 262, 2853, 1989.
70. Ziegler, R.G., Hoover, R.N., Nomura, A.M.Y., West, D.W., Wu, A.H., Pike, M.C., Lake, A.J., Horn-Ross, P.L., Kolonel, L.N., Siiteri, P.K., and Fraumeni, J.F., Jr., Relative weight, weight change, height, and breast cancer risk in Asian-American women, *J. Natl. Cancer Inst.*, 88, 650, 1996.
71. Potischman, N., Swanson, C.A., Siiteri, P.K., and Hoover, R.N., Reversal of relation between body mass and endogenous estrogen concentrations with menopausal status, *J. Natl. Cancer Inst.*, 88, 756, 1996.
72. Woods, M.N., Barnett, J.B., Spiegelman, D., Trail, N., Hertzmark, E., Longcope, C., and Gorbach, S.L., Hormone levels during dietary changes in premenopausal African-American women, *J. Natl. Cancer Inst.*, 88, 1369, 1996.
73. Phillips, R.L., Role of life style and dietary habits in risk of cancer among Seventh-Day Adventists, *Cancer Res.*, 35, 3513, 1975.
74. Miller, A.B., Kelly, A., Choi, N.W., Matthews, V., Morgan, R.W., Munan, L., Burch, J.D., Feather, J., Howe, G.R., and Jain, M., A study of diet and breast cancer, *Am. J. Epidemiol.*, 107, 499, 1978.
75. Lubin, J.H., Blot, W.J., and Burns, P.E., Breast cancer following high dietary fat and protein consumption, *Am. J. Epidemiol.*, 114, 422 (Abstr.), 1981.
76. Graham, S., Marshall, J., Mettlin, C., Rzepka, T., Nemoto, T., and Byers, T., Diet in the epidemiology of breast cancer, *Am. J. Epidemiol.*, 116, 68, 1982.
77. Howe, G.R., Hirohata, T., Hislop, T.G., Iscovich, J.M., Yuan, J.M., Katsouyanni, K., Lubin, F., Marubini, E., Modan, B., and Rohan, T., Dietary factors and risk of breast cancer: combined analysis of 12 case-control studies, *J. Natl. Cancer Inst.*, 82, 561, 1990.
78. Kushi, L.H., Sellers, T.A., Potter, J.D., Nelson, C.L., Munger, R.G., Kaye, S.A., and Folsom, A.R., Dietary fat and postmenopausal breast cancer, *J. Natl. Cancer Inst.*, 84, 1092, 1992.
79. Knekt, P., Albanes, D., Seppanen, R., Aroma, A., Jarvinen, R., Hyvonen, L., Teppo, L., and Pukkala, E., Dietary fat and risk of breast cancer, *Am. J. Clin. Nutr.*, 52, 903, 1990.
80. Willett, W.C., Hunter, D.J., Stampfer, M.J., Colditz, G., Manson, J.E., Spiegelman, D., Rosner, B., Hennekens, C.H., and Speizer, F.E., Dietary fat and fiber in relation to risk of breast cancer, *J. Am. Med. Assoc.*, 268, 2037, 1992.

81. Barrett-Connor, E. and Friedlander, N.J., Dietary fat, calories, and the risk of breast cancer in postmenopausal women: a prospective population-based study, *J. Am. Coll. Nutr.*, 12, 390, 1993.

82. Prentice, R.L., Measurement error and results from analytic epidemiology: dietary fat and breast cancer, *J. Natl. Cancer Inst.*, 88, 1738, 1996.

83. Whittemore, A.S. and Henderson, B.E., Dietary fat and breast cancer: where are we? *J. Natl. Cancer Inst.*, 85, 762, 1993.

84. Willett, W.C. and Hunter, D.J., Vitamin A and cancers of the breast, large bowel, and prostate: epidemiologic evidence, *Nutr. Rev.*, 52, S53, 1994.

85. Katsouyanni, K., Willett, W.C., Trichopoulos, D., Boyle, P., Trichopoulou, A., Vasilaros, S., Papadiamantis, J., and MacMahon, B., Risk of breast cancer among Greek women in relation to nutrient intake, *Cancer*, 61, 181, 1988.

86. Marubini, E., Decarli, A., Costa, A., Mazzoleni, C., Andreoli, C., Barbieri, A., Capitelli, E., Carlotti, M., Cavallo, F., Monferroni, N., Pastorino, U., and Salvini, S., The relationship of dietary intake and serum levels of retinol and β-carotene with breast cancer, *Cancer*, 61, 173, 1988.

87. Zaridze, D., Lifanova, Y., Maximivitch, D., Day, N.E., and Duffy, S.W., Diet, alcohol consumption and reproductive factors in a case-control study of breast cancer in Moscow, *Int. J. Cancer*, 48, 493, 1991.

88. London, S.J., Stein, E.A., Henderson, I.C., Stampfer, M.J., Wood, W.C., Remine, S., Dmochowshi, J.R., Robert, N.J., and Willett, W.C., Carotenoids, retinol and vitamin E and risk of proliferative benign breast disease and breast cancer, *Cancer Causes Control*, 3, 503, 1992.

89. La Vecchia, C., Decarli, A., Franceschi, S., Gentile, A., Negri, E., and Parazzini, F., Dietary factors and the risk of breast cancer, *Nutr. Cancer*, 10, 205, 1987.

90. Rohan, T.E., McMichael, A.J., and Baghurst, P.A., A population-based case-control study of diet and breast cancer in Australia, *Am. J. Epidemiol.*, 128, 478, 1988.

91. Toniolo, P., Riboli, E., Protta, F., Charrel, M., and Cappa, A.P., Calorie-providing nutrients and the risk of breast cancer, *J. Natl. Cancer Inst.*, 81, 278, 1989.

92. Ingram, D.M., Nottage, E., and Roberts, T., The role of diet in the development of breast cancer: a case-control study of patients with breast cancer, benign epithelial hyperplasia and fibrocystic disease of the breast, *Br. J. Cancer*, 64, 187, 1991.

93. Ewertz, M. and Gill, C., Dietary factors and breast-cancer risk in Denmark, *Int. J. Cancer*, 46, 779, 1990.

94. Potischman, N., McCulloch, C.E., Byers, T., Nemoto, T., Stubbe, N., Milch, R., Parker, R., Rasmussen, K.M., Root, M., and Graham, S., Breast cancer and dietary and plasma concentrations of carotenoids and vitamin A, *Am. J. Clin. Nutr.*, 52, 909, 1990.

95. Van't Veer, P., Kolb, C.M., Verhof, P., Kok, F.J., Schouten, E.G., Hermus, R.J., and Sturmans, F., Dietary fiber, β-carotene and breast cancer: results from a case-control study, *Int. J. Cancer*, 45, 825, 1990.

96. Lee, H.P., Gourley, L., Duffy, S.W., Esteve, J., Lee, J., and Day, N.E., Dietary effects on breast cancer risk in Singapore, *Lancet*, 337, 1197, 1991.

97. Graham, S., Hellmann, R., Marshall, J., Freudenheim, J., Vena, J., Swanson, M., Zielezny, M., Nemoto, T., Stubbe, N., and Raimondo, T., Nutritional epidemiology of postmenopausal breast cancer in western New York, *Am. J. Epidemiol.*, 134, 552, 1991.

98. Paganini-Hill, A., Chao, A., Ross, R.K., and Henderson, B.E., Vitamin A, β-carotene and the risk of cancer: a prospective study, *J. Natl. Cancer Inst.*, 79, 443, 1987.

99. Hunter, D.J., Manson, J.E., Colditz, G.A., Stampfer, M.J., Rosner, B., Hennekens, C.H., Speizer, F.E., and Willett, W.C., A prospective study of the intake of vitamins C, E, and A and the risk of breast cancer, *New Engl. J. Med.*, 329, 234, 1993.

100. Graham, S., Zielezny, M., Marshall, J., Priore, R., Freudenheim, J., Brasure, J., Haughey, B., Nasca, P., and Zdeb, M., Diet in the epidemiology of postmenopausal breast cancer in the New York State cohort, *Am. J. Epidemiol.*, 136, 1327, 1992.

101. Negri, E., La Vecchia, C., Franceschi, S., D'Avanzo, B., Talamini, R., Parpinel, M., Ferraroni, M., Filiberti, R., Montella, M., Conti, E., and Decarli, A., Intake of selected micronutrients and the risk of breast cancer, *Int. J. Cancer*, 65, 140, 1996.

102. Wald, N.J., Boreham, J., Hayward, J.L., and Bulbrook, R.D., Plasma retinol, β-carotene and vitamin E levels in relation to the future risk of breast cancer, *Br. J. Cancer*, 49, 321, 1984.

103. Comstock, G.W., Helzlsouer, K.J., and Bush, T.L., Prediagnostic serum levels of carotenoids and vitamin E as related to subsequent cancer in Washington County, Maryland, *Am. J. Clin. Nutr.*, 53, 260S, 1991.

104. Knekt, P., Jarvinen, R., Seppanen, R. Rissanen, A., Aromaa, A., Heinonen, O.P., Albanes, D., Heinonen, M., Pukkala, E., and Teppo, L., Dietary antioxidants and the risk of lung cancer, *Am. J. Epidemiol.*, 134, 471, 1991.

105. The Alpha Tocopherol, Beta Carotene Cancer Prevention Study Group, The effect of vitamin E and beta carotene on the incidence of lung cancer and other cancers in male smokers, *New Engl. J. Med.*, 330, 1029, 1994.

106. Van't Veer, P., Strain, J.J., Fernandez-Crehuet, J., Martin, B.C., Thamm, M., Kardinaal, A.F.M., Kohlmeier, L., Huttunen, J.K., Martin-Moreno, J.M., and Kok, F.J., Tissue antioxidants and postmenopausal breast cancer: the European Community Multicenter Study on Antioxidants, Myocardial Infarction, and Cancer of the breast (EURAMIC), *Cancer Epidemiol. Biomarkers Prev.*, 5, 441, 1996.

107. Rotmensz, N., DePalo, G., Formelli, F., Costa, A., Marubini, E., Campa, T., Crippa, A., Dabesini, G.M., Delle Grottaglie, M., Di Mauro, M.G., Filiberti, A., Gallazi, M., Guzzon, A., Magni, A., Malone, W., Mariani, L., Palvarini, M., Perloff, M., Pizzichetta, M., and Veronesi, U., Long-term tolerability of fenretinamide (4-HPR) in breast cancer patients, *Eur. J. Cancer*, 27, 1127, 1991.

108. Buring, J.E. and Hennekens, C.H., The Women's Health Study: summary of the study design, *J. Myocard. Ischemia*, 4, 27, 1992.

109. Rock, C.L., Saxe, G.A., Ruffin, M.T., August, D.A., and Schottenfeld, D., Carotenoids, vitamin A, and estrogen receptor status in breast cancer, *Nutr. Cancer*, 25, 281, 1996.

110. Freudenheim, J.L., Marshall, J.R., Vena, J.E., Laughlin, R., Brasure, J.R., Swanson, M.K., Nemoto, T., and Graham, S., Premenopausal breast cancer risk and intake of vegetables, fruits and related nutrients, *J. Natl. Cancer Inst.*, 88, 340, 1996.

111. Shamberger, R.J., Tytko, S.A., and Willis, C.E., Antioxidants and cancer. VI. Selenium and age-adjusted human cancer mortality, *Arch. Environ. Health*, 31, 231, 1976.

112. Clark, L.C., The epidemiology of selenium and cancer, *Fed. Proc.*, 44, 2584, 1985.

113. Schrauzer, G.D., White, D.A., and Schneider, C.J., Cancer mortality correlation studies. III. Statistical associations with dietary selenium intake, *Bioinorg. Chem.*, 7, 23, 1977.

114. Basu, T.K., Hill, G.B., Ng, D., Abdi, E., and Temple, N., Serum vitamins A and E, beta-carotene, and selenium in patients with breast cancer, *J. Am. Coll. Nutr.*, 8, 524, 1989.

115. Chaitchik, S., Shenberg, C., Nir-El, Y., and Mantel, M., The distribution of selenium in human blood samples of Israeli population: comparison between normal and breast cancer cases, *Biol. Trace Elem. Res.*, 15, 205, 1988.

116. Hardell, L., Danell, M., Angqvist, C.A., Marklund, S.L., Fredriksson, M., Zakari, A.L., and Kjellgren, A., Levels of selenium in plasma and glutathione peroxidase in erythrocytes and the risk of breast cancer: a case-control study, *Biol. Trace Elem. Res.*, 36, 99, 1993.

117. Van't Veer, P., van der Wielen, R.P., Kok, F.J., Hermus, R.J., and Sturmans, F., Selenium in diet, blood, and toenails in relation to breast cancer: a case-control study, *Am. J. Epidemiol.*, 131, 987, 1990.

118. Van't Veer, P., vann Leer, E.M., Rietdijk, A., Kok, F.J., Schouten, E.G., Hermus, R.J., and Sturmans, F., Combination of dietary factors in relation to breast cancer occurrence, *Int. J. Cancer*, 47, 649, 1991.

119. Gerber, M., Richardson, S., Salkeld, R., and Chappuis, P., Antioxidants in female breast cancer patients, *Cancer Invest.*, 9, 421, 1991.

120. Overvad, K., Gron, P., Langhoff, O., Tarp, U., Foldspang, A., and Thorling, E.B., Selenium in human mammary carcinogenesis: a case-referent study, *Eur. J. Cancer Prev.*, 1, 27, 1991.

121. Pawlowicz, Z., Zachara, B.A., Trafikowska, U., Maciag, A., Marchaluk, E., and Nowicki, A., Blood selenium concentrations and glutathione peroxidase activities in patients with breast cancer and with advanced gastrointestinal cancer, *J. Trace Elem. Electro. Health Dis.*, 5, 275, 1991.

122. Gupta, S., Narang, R., Krishnaswami, K., and Yadav, S., Plasma selenium level in cancer patients, *Ind. J. Cancer*, 31, 192, 1994.

123. Sharma, K., Mittal, D.K., Kesarwani, R.C., Kamboj, V.P., and Chowdery, D., Diagnostic and prognostic significance of serum and tissue trace elements in breast malignancy, *Ind. J. Med. Sci.*, 48, 227, 1994.

124. Hunter, D.J., Morris, J.S., Stampfer, M.J., Colditz, G.A., Speizer, F.E., and Willett, W.C., A prospective study of selenium status and breast cancer risk, *J. Am. Med. Assoc.*, 264, 1128, 1990.

125. van den Brandt, P.A., Goldbohm, R.A., van't Veer, P., Bode, P., Dorant, E., Hermus, R.J., and Sturmans, F., Toenail selenium levels and the risk of breast cancer, *Am. J. Epidemiol.*, 140, 20, 1994.

126. Garland, M., Willett, W.C., Manson, J.E., and Hunter, D.J., Antioxidant micronutrients and breast cancer, *J. Am. Coll. Nutr.*, 12, 400, 1993.
127. Clark, L.C., Combs, G.F., Turnbull, B.W., Slate, E.H., Chalker, D.K., Chow, D., Davis, L.S., Glover, R.A., Graham, G.F., Gross, E.G., Krongrad, A., Lesher, J.L., Park, H.K., Sanders, B.B., Smith, C.L., and Taylor, J.R., Effects of selenium supplementation for cancer prevention in patients with carcinoma of the skin: a randomized controlled trial, *J. Am. Med. Assoc.*, 276, 1957, 1996.
128. Garland, F., Garland, C.F., Gorham, E.D., and Young, J.F., Geographic variation in breast cancer mortality in the United States: a hypothesis involving solar radiation, *Prev. Med.*, 19, 614, 1990.
129. Gorham, E.D., Garland, F.C., and Garland, C.F., Sunlight and breast cancer incidence in the U.S.S.R., *Int. J. Epidemiol.*, 19, 820, 1990.
130. Jacobson, E.A., James, K.A., Newmark, H.L., and Carroll, K.K., Effects of dietary fat, calcium, and vitamin D on growth and mammary tumorigenesis induced by 7,12-dimethylbenz(a)anthracene in female Sprague-Dawley rats, *Cancer Res.*, 49, 6300, 1989.
131. Newmark, H.L., Vitamin D adequacy: a possible relationship to breast cancer, *Adv. Exp. Med. Biol.*, 364, 109, 1994.
132. Simard, A., Vobecky, J., and Vobecky, J.S., Vitamin D deficiency and cancer of the breast: an unprovocative ecological hypothesis, *Can. J. Public Health*, 82, 300, 1991.
133. Christakos, S., Vitamin D and breast cancer, *Adv. Exp. Med. Biol.*, 364, 115, 1994.
134. Colston, K.W., Berger, U., and Coombes, R.C., Possible role for vitamin D in controlling breast cancer cell proliferation, *Lancet*, i, 188, 1989.
135. Colston, K.W., Chander, S.K., Mackay, A.G., and Coombes, R.C., Effects of synthetic vitamin D analogues on breast cancer cell proliferation *in vivo* and *in vitro*, *Biochem. Pharmacol.*, 44, 693, 1992.
136. Pence, B.C. and Dunn, D.M., Vitamin D, cancer, and immunity, *J. Nutr. Immunol.*, 2, 109, 1993.
137. Berger, U., McClelland, R.A., Wilson, P., Greene, G.L., Haussler, M.R., Pike, J.W., Colston, K., Easton, D., and Coombes, R.C., Immunocytochemical determination of estrogen receptor, progesterone receptor, and 1,2-dihydroxyvitamin D_3 receptor in breast cancer and relationship to prognosis, *Cancer Res.*, 51, 239, 1991.
138. Longnecker, M.P., Alcoholic beverage consumption in relation to risk of breast cancer: meta-analysis and review, *Cancer Causes Control*, 5, 73, 1994.
139. Howe, G., Rohan, T., Decarli, A., Iscovitch, J., Kaldor, J., Katsouyanni, K., Marubini, E., Miller, A., Riboli, E., Toniolo, P., and Trichopoulos, D., The association between alcohol and breast cancer risk: evidence from the combined analysis of six dietary case-control studies, *Int. J. Cancer*, 47, 707, 1991.
140. Rosenberg, L., Metzger, L.S., and Palmer, J.R., Alcohol consumption and risk of breast cancer: a review of the epidemiological evidence, *Epidemiol. Rev.*, 15, 133, 1993.
141. Roth, H.D., Levy, P.S., Shi, L., and Post, E., Alcoholic beverages and breast cancer: some observations on published case-control studies, *J. Clin. Epidemiol.*, 47, 207, 1994.

142. Williams, R.R. and Horm, J.W., Association of cancer sites with tobacco and alcohol consumption and socioeconomic status of patients: interview study from the Third National Cancer Survey, *J. Natl. Cancer Inst.*, 58, 525, 1977.

143. Rosenberg, L., Slone, D., Shapiro, S., Kaufman, D.W., Helmrich, S.P., Miettinen, O.S., Stolley, P.D., Levy, M., Rosenshein, N.B., Schottenfeld, D., and Engle, R.L., Jr., Breast cancer and alcoholic-beverage consumption, *Lancet*, i, 267, 1982.

144. Adami, H.-O., Lund, E., Bergstrom, R., and Meirik, O., Cigarette smoking, alcoholic beverage consumption, and risk of breast cancer in young women, *Br. J. Cancer*, 58, 832, 1988.

145. Byers, T. and Funch, D.P., Alcohol and breast cancer (letter), *Lancet*, 1, 799, 1982.

146. Harris, R.E. and Wynder, E.L., Breast cancer and alcohol consumption: a study in weak associations, *J. Am. Med. Assoc.*, 259, 2867, 1988.

147. Meara, J., McPherson, K., Roberts, M., Jones, L., and Vessey, M., Alcohol, cigarette smoking and breast cancer, *Br. J. Cancer*, 60, 70, 1989.

148. Rosenberg, L., Palmer, J.R., Miller, D.R., Clarke, E.A., and Shapiro, S., A case-control study of alcoholic beverage consumption and breast cancer, *Am. J. Epidemiol.*, 131, 6, 1990.

149. Longnecker, M., Berlin, J.A., Orza, M.J., and Chalmers, T.C., A meta-analysis of alcohol consumption in relation to risk of breast cancer, *J. Am. Med. Assoc.*, 260, 652, 1988.

150. Martin-Moreno, J.M., Boyle, P., Gorgojo, L., Willett, W.C., Gonzalez, J., Villar, F., and Maissoneuve, P., Alcoholic beverage consumption and risk of breast cancer in Spain, *Cancer Causes Control*, 4, 345, 1993.

151. Katsouyanni, K., Trichopoulou, A., Stuver, S., Vassilaros, S., Papadiamantis, Y., Bournas, N., Skarpou, N., Mueller, N., and Trichopoulos, D., Ethanol and breast cancer: an association that may be both confounded and causal, *Int. J. Cancer*, 58, 356, 1994.

152. Holmberg, L., Ohlander, E.M., Byers, T., Zack, M., Wolk, A., Bergstrom, R., Bergkvist, L., Thurfjell, E., Bruce, A., and Adami, H.O., Diet and breast cancer risk: results from a population-based, case-control study in Sweden, *Arch. Intern. Med.*, 154, 1805, 1994.

153. Smith, S.J., Deacon, J.M., and Chilvers, C.E., Alcohol, smoking, passive smoking, and caffeine in relation to breast cancer risk in young women, *Br. J. Cancer*, 70, 112, 1994.

154. Reichman, M.E., Judd, J.T., Longcope, C., Schatzkin, A., Clevidence, B.A., Nair, P.P., Campbell, W.S., and Taylor, P.R., Effects of alcohol consumption on plasma and urinary hormone concentrations in premenopausal women, *J. Natl. Cancer Inst.*, 85, 722, 1993.

155. Dorgan, J.F., Reichman, M.E., Judd, J.T., Brown, C., Longcope, C., Schatzkin, A., Campbell, W.S., Franz, C., Kahle, L., and Taylor, P.R., The relation of reported alcohol ingestion to plasma levels of estrogens and androgens in premenopausal women, *Cancer Causes Control*, 5, 53, 1994.

156. Kurzer, M.S., Diet, estrogen and cancer, *Contemp. Nutr.*, 17, 1, 1992.

157. Adlercreutz, H., Mousavi, Y., Clark, J., Hockerstedt, K., Hamalainen, E., Wahala, K., Makela, T., and Hase, T., Dietary phytoestrogens and cancer: *in vitro* and *in vivo* studies, *J. Steroid Biochem. Mol. Biol.*, 41, 331, 1992.

158. Messina, M., Persky, V., Setchell, K.D.R., and Barnes, S., Soy intake and cancer risk: a review of *in vitro* and *in vivo* data, *Nutr. Cancer*, 21, 113, 1994.

159. Lee, H.P., Gourley, L., Duffy, S.W., Esteve, J., Lee, J., and Day, N.E., Risk factors for breast cancer by age and menopausal status: a case-control study in Singapore, *Cancer Causes Control*, 3, 313, 1992.

160. Wu, A.H., Ziegler, R.G., Horn-Ross, P.L., Nomura, A.M.Y., West, D.W., Kolonel, L.N., Rosenthal, J.F., Hoover, R.N., and Pike, M.C., Tofu and risk of breast cancer in Asian-Americans, *Cancer Epidemiol. Biomarkers Prev.*, 5, 901, 1996.

161. Thompson, L.U., Robb, P., Serraino, M., and Cheung, F., Mammalian lignan production from various foods, *Nutr. Cancer*, 16, 43, 1991.

162. Phipps, W.R., Martini, M.C., Lampe, J.W., Slavin, J.L., and Kurzer, M.S., Effect of flaxseed ingestion on the menstrual cycle: possible relevance to diet-related breast cancer risk, *Ann. Meet. Soc. Gynecol. Invest.*, 1993.

163. Goldbohm, R.A., Bertog, M.G., Brants, H.A., van Poppel, G., and van den Brandt, P.A., Consumption of black tea and cancer risk: a prospective cohort study, *J. Natl. Cancer Inst.*, 88, 93, 1996.

164. Lubin, J.H., Burns, P.E., Blot, W.J., Ziegler, R.G., Lees, A.W., and Fraumeni, J.F., Dietary factors and breast cancer risk, *Int. J. Cancer*, 28, 685, 1981.

165. Kinlen, L.J., Meat and fat consumption and cancer mortality: a study of strict religious orders in Britain, *Lancet*, 1, 946, 1982.

166. Phillips, R.L. and Snowdon, D.A., Association of meat and coffee use with cancers of the large bowel, breast and prostate among Seventh-Day Adventists: preliminary results, *Cancer Res.*, 43, 2403S, 1983.

167. Zemla, B., The role of selected dietary elements in breast cancer risk among native and migrant populations in Poland, *Nutr. Cancer*, 6, 187, 1984.

168. Mills, P.K., Annegers, J.F., and Phillips, R.L., Animal product consumption and subsequent fatal breast cancer risk among Seventh-Day Adventists, *Am. J. Epidemiol.*, 127, 440, 1988.

169. Van den Brandt, P.A., Goldbohm, R.A., van Loon, A.J.K., and Kok, F.J., Cross-sectional vs. longitudinal investigations of the diet–cancer relation, *Epidemiology*, 1, 402, 1990.

170. Vatten, L.J., Salvall, K., and Laken, E.B., Frequency of meat and fish intake and risk of breast cancer in a prospective study of 14,500 Norwegian women, *Int. J. Cancer*, 46, 12, 1990.

171. Toniolo, P., Riboli, E., Shore, R.E., and Pasternack, B.S., Consumption of meat, animal products, protein, and fat and risk of breast cancer: a prospective cohort study in New York, *Epidemiology*, 5, 391, 1994.

172. Landa, M.C., Frago, N., and Tres, A., Diet and the risk of breast cancer in Spain, *Eur. J. Cancer Prev.*, 3, 313, 1994.

173. Gaard, M., Tretli, S., and Laken, E.B., Dietary fat and the risk of breast cancer: a prospective study of 25,892 Norwegian women, *Int. J. Cancer*, 63, 13, 1995.

174. Matos, E.L., Thomas, D.B., Sobel, N., and Vuota, D., Breast cancer in Argentina: case-control study with special reference to meat eating habits, *Neoplasma*, 38, 357, 1991.

175. Boyd, N.F., Martin, L.J., Noffel, M., Lockwood, G.A., and Trichler, D.L., A meta-analysis of studies of dietary fat and breast cancer risk, *Br. J. Cancer*, 68, 627, 1993.

176. Ronco, A., DeStefani, E., Mendilaharsu, M., and Deneo-Pellegrini, H., Meat, fat and risk of breast cancer: a case-control study from Uruguay, *Int. J. Cancer*, 65, 328, 1996.

177. Ito, N., Hasegawa, R., Sano, M., Tamano, S., Esumi, H., Takayama, S., and Sugimura, T., A new colon and mammary carcinogen in cooked food, 2-amino-1-methyl-6-phenylimidazo[4,5-*b*]pyridine (PhIP), *Carcinogenesis*, 12, 1503, 1991.

178. Kato, T., Migita, H., Ohgaki, H., Sato, T., Takayama, S., and Sugimura, T., Induction of tumors in the Zymbal gland, oral cavity, colon, skin, and mammary gland of F344 rats by a mutagenic compound, 2-amino-3,4-dimethylimidazo[4,5-*f*]quinoline, *Carcinogenesis*, 10, 601, 1989.

179. Tanaka, T., Barnes, W.S., Williams, G.M., and Weisburger, J.H., Multipotential carcinogenicity of the fried food mutagen 2-amino-3-methylimidaz[4,5-*f*]quinoline in rats, *Jpn. J. Cancer Res.*, 76, 570, 1985.

180. Snyderwine, E.G., Some perspectives on the nutritional aspects of breast cancer research: food-derived heterocyclic amines as etiologic agents in human mammary cancer, *Cancer*, 74, 1070, 1994.

181. Lubin, F. and Ron, E., Consumption of methylxanthine-containing beverages and the risk of breast cancer, *Cancer Lett.*, 53, 81, 1990.

182. Phelps, H.M. and Phelps, C.E., Caffeine ingestion and breast cancer. A negative correlation, *Cancer*, 61, 1051, 1988.

183. Folsom, A.R., McKenzie, D.R., Bisgard, K.M., Kushi, L.H., and Sellers, T.A., No association between caffeine intake and postmenopausal breast cancer incidence in the Iowa Women's Health Study, *Am. J. Epidemiol.*, 138, 380, 1993.

184. Millikan, R., DeVoto, E., Newman, B., and Savitz, D., Studying environmental influences and breast cancer risk: suggestions for an integrated population-based approach, *Breast Cancer Res. Treat.*, 35, 79, 1995.

185. Falck, F., Jr., Ricci, A., Jr., Wolff, M.S., Godbold, J., and Deckers, P., Pesticides and polychlorinated biphenyl residues in human breast lipids and their relation to breast cancer, *Arch. Environ. Health*, 47, 143, 1992.

186. Wolff, M.S., Toniolo, P.G., Lee, E.W., Rivera, M., and Dubin, N., Blood levels of organochlorine residues and risk of breast cancer, *J. Natl. Cancer Inst.*, 85, 648, 1993.

187. Hunter, D.J. and Willett, W.C., Nutrition and breast cancer, *Cancer Causes Control*, 7, 56, 1996.

CHAPTER 3

NUTRITION AND CANCER OF THE CERVIX

CONTENTS

I. GENERAL PATHOLOGY AND STATISTICS

Although the cervical cancer incidence rates have decreased in the United States in the past 40 years, this cancer site remains a significant problem in the lower socioeconomic strata, as well as in other parts of the world.[1] Cervical cancer accounts for about 2% of all newly diagnosed cancers in women and 2% of all cancer-related deaths.[2] The Papanicolaou cytologic test (Pap smear) assesses for abnormal cells shed from the endocervix and has drastically reduced the incidence of cervical cancer deaths.

The Cervical Intraepithelial Neoplasia (CIN) classification for cervical precancers is as follows:[3]

Human papillomavirus	CIN I
Mild dysplasia	
Moderate dysplasia	CIN II
Severe dysplasia	CIN III
Carcinoma *in situ*	

There is evidence to support a continuum or progression from human papillomavirus (HPV) infection to dysplasia and subsequently to the development of carcinoma. The majority of cervical cancers are preceded by a precancerous lesion which sheds abnormal cells. Relatively indistinct boundaries are noted where premalignant changes are occurring. Some changes may spontaneously regress, but the risk of progression to cancer increases with severity. HPV infection and dysplasia nearly always arises at the squamocolumnar junction (transformation zone). High-risk HPV types (especially 16 and 18) are found most often in the higher grade precursors. Progression to invasive cancer, if it occurs, may take from several months to many years.[4,5]

Squamous cell carcinoma occurs at a peak age incidence of 40–45 years. Grossly, it may be fungating, ulcerating, or infiltrative. Histologically, it may be large cell keratinizing, large cell nonkeratinizing, or small cell squamous. Cervical adenocarcinoma comprises 3–7% of cervical carcinomas. This is thought to arise from the endocervical glands. They look grossly and behave like squamous cell lesions but arise in a slightly older age group. There may be an association with HPV similar to squamous cell carcinoma. Adenosquamous carcinoma can also occur, which has a poorer prognosis than squamous cell alone.

Cervical small-cell undifferentiated carcinoma (neuroendocrine) comprises less than 5% of cervical carcinomas. Histologically, it is similar to small cell carcinoma of the lung, with early metastasis and high mortality. Cervical cancer is staged as follows:[6]

Stage 0. Carcinoma *in situ* (CIN III).
Stage I. Carcinoma confined to cervix.
    Ia. Preclinical carcinoma, i.e., diagnosed only by microscopy but showing:
        Ia1. Minimal microscopic invasion of stroma (minimally invasive carcinoma).
        Ia2. Microscopic invasion of stroma of less than 5 mm in depth (microinvasive carcinoma).
    Ib. Histologically invasive carcinoma of the cervix that is greater than stage Ia2.
Stage II. Carcinoma extends beyond the cervix but not into the pelvic wall. Carcinoma involves the vagina but not the lower third.
Stage III. Carcinoma has extended into pelvic wall. On rectal examination, there is no cancer-free space between the tumor and the pelvic wall. The tumor involves the lower third of the vagina.

Stage IV. Carcinoma has extended beyond the true pelvis or has involved the mucosa of the bladder or rectum. This stage obviously includes those with metastatic dissemination.*

With current methods of treatment, there is a 5-year survival rate of about 80–90% with stage I, 75% with stage II, 35% with stage III, and 10–15% with stage IV disease.[7] As stated previously, the widespread use of the Pap smear has significantly decreased mortality from this disease in developed countries.

II. POPULATION GENETICS AND MARKERS FOR RISK

A. Human Papillomavirus

Although there is overwhelming evidence that infection by the HPV and subsequent integration into the host genome is important in the development of cervical cancer, a number of other genetic factors have been studied as well. The genetics of cervical cancer has been reviewed by both Taylor et al.[8] and Baker,[9] and no well-defined familial or somatic genetic lesions appear to be prominent in the etiology of this disease, except for interactions involving the genome of HPV with host DNA. HPV appears to be the most conspicuous marker for risk of cervical neoplasia. Only 15% of cervical cancers appear to be negative for HPV, but even with over 85% positive for the presence of the virus, it seems that infection is neither necessary nor sufficient alone to cause cervical cancer. The evidence linking HPV infection is compelling for the following reasons: most cervical dysplasia is associated with HPV infection with 1 of the 60 types discovered so far; integrated HPV DNA has been seen in dysplastic lesions as well as in invasive lesions from the same patient; certain HPV types can immortalize keratinocytes in culture; and finally, HPV types 16 and 18 can produce the viral transformation proteins E6 and E7, which bind to both the *p53* protein and *Rb*, resulting in the promotion of deregulated cellular proliferation.[8]

B. Oncogenes

Several oncogenes have been examined for their role in the molecular genetics of cervical cancer. Analysis of members of the *ras* gene family has shown only codon 12 of the c-Ha-*ras* gene to be mutated in cervical cancer.[10] In contrast, overexpression of the p21 *ras* protein has been detected in over 52% of cervical tumors.[11] Studies of expression only of c-Ha-*ras* have demonstrated this phenomenon in 12% of tumors examined, but that this was more

* From Cotran, R.S., Kumar, V., and Robbins, S.L., *Robbins Pathologic Basis of Disease*, 5th ed., W.B. Saunders, Philadelphia, 1994, 1052. With permission.

common with nodal metastasis.[12] Thus, Taylor et al.[8] concluded that mutational activation of *ras* genes may only play a minor role in the development of this tumor.

Both overexpression and amplification of the c-*myc* oncogene have been investigated in cervical cancer. Overexpression of *myc* has been found in about 40% of tumors analyzed in several studies,[13–15] and this overexpression has corresponded to advanced-stage disease and poor survival. c-*myc* amplification has also been demonstrated[13, 16, 17] and is also correlated with advanced-stage disease.[13] Taylor et al.[8] hypothesized that c-*myc* appears to act late in the course of cervical cancer development as a progression factor.

The epithelial growth factor receptor (EGF-R) has been found to be overexpressed in 100% of cervical tumors examined by Berchuck et al.,[18] and Pfeiffer et al.[19] demonstrated increased numbers of EGF-R in tumors and correlated them with metastatic disease. Her-2/neu expression was found in 38% of cervical tumors,[20] however, with overexpression seen in only 3% of tumors.[18] Chromosome 1 rearrangement and loss of heterozygosity at 3p and 17p have also been documented in cervical tumors, but the specific genes involved have not been identified, except in the case of *p53*.[21–24] The *p53* tumor suppressor gene has probably been the most extensively studied genetic locus in cervical carcinoma, but mutation has been found to be uncommon in this tumor. It appears to be limited primarily to those tumors that are HPV-negative, suggesting an alternative molecular mechanism of transformation.[25–27] Conversely, HPV-positive tumors are found to have *p53* mutations only rarely. It is speculated that the reason for this appears to lie in the fact that the HPV E6 protein binds to the *p53* protein, thus rendering the cell *p53*-negative.[28]

C. Family History

In summary, there does not appear to be a strong case for the involvement of specific genetic lesions in the etiology of most cervical cancer. The major risk factor from an epidemiologic standpoint, as well as a molecular one, appears to be the interaction of the HPV genome with that of the host cell. The oncogene mutations found in cervical cancer may represent an alternative pathway of transformation, or they may be late events in the multistage tumor development process. No published studies have examined the possibility of familial cervical cancers. Only anecdotal reports have identified potential familial clustering of cervical carcinoma.[29] Lynch et al.[29] concluded that these reports of multiple cases in sisters were difficult to interpret, considering the high population frequency of this disease. Only one case-control study done in Malmo, Sweden, demonstrated the possibility of hereditary influences. Kullander[30] reported that cervical cancer was seven times more likely to occur in patients' sisters and mothers than in a control group taken from the families of the partners of the affected women. Therefore, it appears that the most compelling genetic event which occurs in cervical cancer is HPV infection, and this does not appear to be a familial phenomenon.

III. GENERAL EPIDEMIOLOGY OF CERVICAL CANCER

A. Human Papillomavirus

Generally, infection with HPV is considered as the major cause of cervical cancer. A number of epidemiological studies of cases and controls have demonstrated relative risks for invasive cervical cancer of between 4 and 40.[31] Thus, the great majority of women with cervical and/or squamous intraepithelial lesions have detectable HPV DNA, compared to a consistently lower percentage of control women.[31] Many types of HPV exist, and a number have been associated with cancer, but by most reports HPV type 16 is the most important cancer-associated type, along with types 18, 31, and 45.[32] From what is known about HPV and cervical neoplasia, it appears that the HPV infection (confirmed by the presence of HPV DNA) precedes and even predicts incident cervical neoplasia.[31] A recent study by Burger et al.[33] tested the hypothesis that differences in survival among cervical cancer patients were associated with a difference in HPV DNA types. In a historical cohort of 291 with all stages of cervical carcinoma, Burger et al.[33] found that the presence of HPV type 18 DNA is an independent prognostic factor in patients treated for early-stage cervical cancer and is predictive for risk of recurrence. However, an editorial in the same journal in which the above article was published refers to a National Institutes of Health consensus conference on cervical cancer in April 1996 in which the participants recommended against a treatment policy that plans radical surgery and pelvic radiation therapy.[34] Therefore, the use of HPV DNA typing in the management of patients is still only a research technique.

Other issues relevant to the involvement of HPV in cervical neoplasia are in two reports which examined male sexual behavior and its role in female cervical cancer in both Spain and Colombia. Bosch et al.[35] evaluated the role of men's sexual behavior and the presence of HPV DNA in the penis on the development of cervical cancer in their sexual partners in Spain, a low-risk area for cervical cancer. They found that the presence of HPV DNA in the husbands' penis conveyed a fivefold risk of cervical cancer to their wives and that this risk was strongly associated with type 16 and related to the number of extramarital sex partners. The authors concluded that men who have multiple sex partners and/or who are HPV 16 carriers may be vectors of high risk for cervical cancer in their wives. In contrast, another study of male sexual behavior as a risk factor for cervical cancer examined the presence of penile HPV DNA on risk in an area of Colombia that has a high incidence of cervical cancer.[36] However, the only significant risk factors identified were limited education and the presence of *Chlamydia trachomatis* antibodies in husbands. Neither the presence of HPV DNA in the penis nor the number of lifetime female sex partners was associated with the risk of cervical cancer. These authors concluded that the presence of HPV DNA in the penis of adult men is a poor reflection of lifetime exposure to HPV and that the role of *C. trachomatis* in cervical cancer needs further investigation.[36] Interestingly, an earlier study also assessed the impact of women's sexual activity and their subsequent risk for developing cervical cancer.[37] The study reported the sexual history of a group of white middle-class American women and concluded that 72.3% should be considered at high risk for developing cervical cancer and its precursors and should be screened regularly for this disease. Along the same lines, Viaque and Fenollar[38] reported in an ecological study of the distribution of cervical cancer in Spain that the mortality from this cancer in urban areas supported the hypothesis that cervical cancer is more frequent because women in urban areas demonstrate greater promiscuity and relaxation of sexual behaviors.

B. Other Risk Factors

Other investigations have examined a number of interesting and somewhat unusual associations with risk for cervical cancer. Gardner et al.[39] investigated the practice of douching and its relationship to risk and concluded that frequent douching may be a risk factor in that the practice alters the vaginal chemical environment, thus possibly making the cervix more susceptible to pathologic change. The presence of *Trichomonas vaginalis* infections has also been assessed as a potential risk factor. Gram et al.[40] examined the temporal relationship between cervical infection with *T. vaginalis* and HPV and the incidence rate of cervical intraepithelial neoplasia in Norwegian women. They confirmed that HPV was a causal factor but that there may also be an association between *T. vaginalis* infection and cervical neoplasia as well. Subsequent reports from Zhang et al.[41,42] found that there is an association between *T. vaginalis* infection and the risk of cervical cancers, but that this accounts for only 2% of cases.[41] Zhang et al.[42] also pursued this hypothesis in a population of Chinese women in a prospective study and found that there might be an association between *T. vaginalis* and cervical carcinoma, but it would only account for 4–5% of cervical cancer in Chinese women.

Smoking has also been hypothesized as a risk factor for cervical cancer; however, in most studies not adjusted for the presence of HPV, the relative risks have been only about twofold (see Shiffman et al.[31] for a thorough review). In the more definitive reports which have adjusted for HPV status, the influence of smoking drops to almost null.[31] This confounding control has been addressed by Phillips and Smith,[43] and they concluded that the observed independent effect of smoking on cervical cancer was due to residual confounding, even after adjusting for the role of HPV infection.

The use of oral contraceptives and risk for cervical cancer has long been of interest, but the interpretation of these studies is complex due to the potential confounding by sexual behavior and screening practices.[31] A number of recent case-control studies have been summarized by Shiffman et al.,[31] although these results have not been adjusted for HPV infection. These authors concluded that the majority of studies indicated that long-term users are at excess risk, even after adjustment for sexual and social factors. A recent large study conducted by the World Health Organization[44] reported a risk of 2.2 for cervical cancer in women who were users for 8 or more years. There has also been recent interest in the possible interaction between oral contraceptive use and HPV. Two recent studies have found an elevated risk of invasive cervical carcinoma among HPV-positive women who had used oral contraceptives.[45,46] It has been speculated that oral contraceptive use may promote the activity of HPV after infection has occurred.

In summary, the most compelling risk factor for the development of cervical cancer appears to be exposure to the HPV of either DNA type 16 or 18. Many of the other risk factors discussed here decline in significance when adjusted for HPV positivity. A number of these other risk factors such as use of oral contraceptives, sexual practices, and infection with other sexually transmitted diseases all could be considered as surrogate variables for promiscuity and subsequent increased probability of exposure to and infection with HPV. Therefore, it can be concluded that the overwhelming influence on whether or not a woman gets cervical cancer stems from her probability of contracting the HPV infection. This is supported by a number of studies of sexual behavior which link age at first sexual intercourse and invasive cervical cancer. It has been shown in a variety of case-control studies that women who become sexually active before age 16 have a twofold increased risk.[31] It has also been demonstrated that the risk of cervical cancer is influenced by the number of sexual partners over the life span, again reflecting the association with the probability of HPV exposure and infection.

IV. VITAMIN A AND CAROTENOIDS

Nutritional influences on the development of cervical cancer have long been of interest. Many nutrients have been studied for a possible relationship to cervical neoplasia, especially the carotenoids and vitamin A, because of their known effects on control of differentiation in squamous epithelium (Table 3.1). The majority of reports have found no association between the intake of preformed vitamin A and the risk of cervical dysplasia, *in situ* cancer, or invasive disease (for an excellent review, see Potischman[1]). Many of the earlier studies, including both serologic studies and dietary intake studies, concluded that there was no relationship between vitamin A and cervical neoplasia.[1] One study by

Table 3.1   Case-Control Studies of Vitamins and Cervical Cancer

Nutrient/Type of Study	Association with Risk	Reference
Vitamin A/dietary	Inverse	47, 48
Carotenoids/dietary	Inverse	47, 49–54
	Direct	58
	No association	49, 55–57
Carotenoids/serologic	Inverse	Reviewed in 1
	Inverse, stage IV disease only	62
	No association	59–61
Vitamin C/dietary	Inverse	48, 50, 52–54, 58, 64
	No association	55–57
Vitamin C/serologic	Inverse	64, 65
	No association	66
Vitamin E/serologic	Inverse with higher grade lesions	68, 69
	Inverse; prospective study	70
Folate/dietary	Inverse	48, 81, 82
	No association	50, 52, 53, 55, 57
Folate/serologic	Inverse	81
	Inverse with advanced disease	64
	No association	83, 84

Wylie-Rosett et al.[47] reported lower vitamin A intake associated with cervical cancer but only used a 3-day diet record to assess intake, now considered a somewhat inadequate assessment. However, a more recent study of Alabama women investigated an association of nutritional factors with cervical dysplasia in a case-control study[48] using a 24-hour dietary recall to assess nutritional intake. Vitamin A intake showed a significantly increased risk at the lowest quartile of intake compared to the highest quartile with an odds ratio of 2.2. There was also a significant trend for risk with decreasing intake of vitamin A.[48] Nevertheless, the preponderance of the evidence does not demonstrate a strong relationship between vitamin A and cervical cancer at any stage.

Many of the earlier dietary studies investigated case-control differences in relation to intake of carotenoids. However, these studies as well were mixed in their results. Seven studies of dietary intake of carotenoids showed that cases had lower intakes than controls,[47, 49–54] and these were in relation to cervical dysplasia specifically,[47, 54] in situ cancer,[50] and invasive cervical cancer.[49, 51–53] In contrast, four additional studies reported no differences between cases and controls, whether it be for risk for dysplasia,[49] in situ cancer,[55, 56] or invasive cervical cancer.[57] Only one study[58] showed a higher intake of carotenoids as beta-carotene among cases compared to controls. Serologic studies showed similar distribution, with more studies reporting serum carotenoids being lower in cases than controls. However, as seen with the dietary intake studies, there were also four studies which demonstrated no differences. However, three of these studies have been criticized[59–61] because they had such small sample sizes among cases (less than 32 cases[1]). The most recent report available on the relationship between cervical cancer and serological markers of nutritional status was performed on a Latin American population.[62] This study found lower alpha- and beta-carotene values only among those women with stage IV disease and cautioned that there may be confounding disease effects of these nutrients in studies of serum markers and cervical cancer. In summary, of all the data on carotenoids, Potischman[1] has concluded in her review that although there is some indication that carotenoid intake and status may be important in cervical neoplasia, the results are far from consistent.

Very recently, a Phase II study used p.o. beta-carotene to treat CIN I and II.[63] The data indicated that a large percentage of patients would respond clinically to p.o. beta-carotene supplementation, as determined with cytology, colposcopy, and/or biopsies. The authors stated that ongoing prospective randomized studies will compare the efficacy of beta-carotene against an untreated control arm.[63]

V. VITAMIN C

Most studies of vitamin C (as ascorbic acid), whether dietary or serologic, seemed to be associated with a reduction in risk for cervical neoplasia. In terms of dietary intake of vitamin C, this nutrient was found to be protective against cervical dysplasia, in *in situ* as well as in invasive cancer.[50, 52–54, 58, 64] However, three studies found no differences in *in situ* or invasive cervical cancer risk.[55–57] There have only been three serologic studies to date, and two found a difference between serum ascorbate levels and cervical cancer risk[64, 65] and one did not.[66] Interestingly, two of the dietary studies only found a protective effect with vitamin C intake among women who were smokers,[56,57] which is not surprising considering the association between smoking and this disease (for review, see Shiffman et al.[31]) and the well-known increased requirement for vitamin C among smokers.[67] In the most recent study of nutritional factors and cervical dysplasia, Liu et al.[48] also reported that increased risk was associated with lower intakes for vitamin C compared to the highest intake level. These data collectively suggest that higher intakes of vitamin C may be protective for cervical neoplasia and that the effects may be even more important in those women who choose to smoke. However, the difficulty associated with the serologic assessment of vitamin C status due to special handling requirements for the blood samples may limit the value of this means of assessing associations.[1]

VI. VITAMIN E

Vitamin E has not been studied as extensively in terms of cervical neoplasia, and most studies have been serologic investigations.[68–70] Only one of these studies was prospective in design,[70] and this reported that higher levels of vitamin E in serum were associated with a reduced risk of developing cervical cancer. This effect persisted after exclusion of cancers which developed within 2 years of the blood collection, suggesting that the effect was not a consequence of the disease process. Two other serologic studies found lower levels of vitamin E to be associated with a higher grade lesion, and even lower concentrations were seen in those with invasive cancers.[68,69] In summary, the studies of vitamin E and cervical cancer showed mixed results with no clear-cut conclusion that could be drawn.

VII. FOLATE

The case for folate in the etiology of cervical cancer is probably stronger than for any other nutrient studied. Since 1977, several reports have indicated an increased incidence of cervical cancer among oral contraceptive users.[71–74] An early study reported that there were morphologic similarities between megaloblastic anemia and those features present in the cervical cells of oral contraceptive users.[75] Supplementation with 10 mg daily of oral folate improved the cervical dysplasia associated with oral contraceptive use.[76] This suggested that cervical epithelium may be sensitive to folate status. However, a more extensive trial of folate supplementation[77] in a group of cervical dysplasia patients failed to demonstrate improvement in biopsy status at the end of the 6-month trial. This lack of an effect of folate supplementation has now been attributed to misclassification of megaloblastic features as dysplasia.[78] There has also been shown to be an association between HPV type 16 prevalence and lowered folate status, which suggests that folate status may be linked with HPV infection and not with dysplastic progression.[79] According to Butterworth,[78] the prevailing view is that folate deficiency is not carcinogenic alone but acts as a cocarcinogenic factor in the presence of other oncologic events, such as may be the case with HPV type 16 or 18 infection. It has been demonstrated in the established cervical carcinoma cell line SW756[80] that the genome of HPV-18 is integrated at a single site on chromosome 12, which is the same location as a folate-sensitive fragile site and which may have facilitated the incorporation of the HPV genome.[80] There is also evidence of involvement of folate deficiency in other cancers or premalignant conditions of the esophagus, lung, colon, and hematopoietic system.[78]

Dietary studies of folate status and cervical cancer have yielded interesting trends. There appears to be more of an association of folate status with dysplasia rather than with more advanced *in situ* or invasive lesions.[1] Van Eenwyk et al.[81] reported reduced risk associated with higher folate levels measured in dietary intake, serum, and red blood cells. McPherson[82] performed a dietary analysis on women with cervical dysplasia and found that the cases had lower folate intake than controls. Recently, Liu et al.[48] have also reported from their case-control study in Alabama that for folate, increased risk for cervical dysplasia was found in the second highest quartile compared with the highest quartile, with an odds ratio of 2.0. Most other studies of dietary folate intake have reported no effects of folate intake and risk for either *in situ*[50,55] or invasive cervical cancer.[52,53,57] However, Butterworth et al.[83] found no effect for serum or red blood cell folate after adjustment for other risk factors, but did report the significant interaction with HPV infection and folate status. Among studies of folate status and more advanced disease, only one study has reported that cases had lower plasma folate levels than controls.[64] However, Potischman et al.[84] in a case-control study of serum folate levels and invasive cervical cancer found no difference between cases and controls.

VIII. OTHER NUTRIENTS

Other nutrients which have been studied in relationship to cervical cancer include riboflavin, selenium, serum lipid status, and the consumption of fruits and vegetables. Liu et al.[48] in their Alabama study of nutritional factors and cervical dysplasia also reported that riboflavin showed increased risk at the two lower quartiles of intake. Another author has examined selenium status and its association with cervical cancer risk. Slattery et al.[56] examined dietary intake of a number of micronutrients, including selenium, in a case-control study in Utah and found no association between selenium intake and cervical cancer risk. In a study of the associations between cervical cancer and serological markers of nutritional status in Latin America, an inverse trend for cholesterol and triglyceride concentrations was observed, suggesting a clinical effect of cervical cancer on blood lipids.[62] A single study has associated pork intake and HPV-related disease.[85] Schneider et al.[85] reported that international correlations suggest that pork intake is positively associated with incidence of cervical cancer, a disease we also know to be related to HPV. The authors[85] suggest that pork meat or dietary factors associated with pork meat consumption may be involved in the development of HPV-related diseases such as cervical cancer.

IX. GENERAL CONCLUSIONS, SUMMARY, AND IMPLICATIONS

There is currently overwhelming evidence that infection by HPV is the key risk factor in the development of cervical cancer. Other genetic risk factors predisposing to the disease have only a minor role to play or they have yet to be identified. Thus, the risk for cervical cancer is more dependent on environmental sexual exposures to HPV than to any predisposing familial susceptibility to this cancer. It is currently unknown whether some individuals are more easily infected with HPV than others in terms of host susceptibility for the virus. Most other factors such as use of oral contraceptives, sexual practices, and infection with other sexually transmitted diseases should all be considered as surrogate variables for promiscuous behavior and, therefore, for increased probability of exposure to and infection with HPV.

The relationship between vitamin A, the carotenoids, and cervical cancer shows some indication that the intake of these nutrients and the overall vitamin A status of the individual may be important in cervical neoplasia, but the large body of data are far from consistent, so no concrete recommendations can be made. Higher intakes of vitamin C may be protective, but the effect may only be evident in women who smoke and, therefore, have higher daily requirements for vitamin C. No conclusions can be drawn for the role of vitamin E in cervical cancer risk. The epidemiology of nutrition and cervical cancer has also recently been reviewed by Potischman and Brinton.[86]

The case for folate is probably more compelling than for any other nutrient studied in association with cervical cancer. The association between folate status and cervical dysplasia is most convincing, although there are some negative studies. Most interesting is the potential connection between folate status and HPV infection, and more research is needed on the intake of folate and susceptibility to HPV infection following exposure.

In summary, there are no strong compelling nutritional factors which are predictors for cervical cancer, with the possible exception of folate. The overwhelming etiological agent for cervical cancer appears to be HPV infection, which can be somewhat prevented by more prudent sexual practices. However, the area of nutritional modulation of HPV host susceptibility is a research area which needs more attention, as the studies with folate have revealed. There are always permissive host factors to be considered in any viral infection, and that is where nutrition may have its greatest impact in this disease.

REFERENCES

1. Potischman, N., Nutritional epidemiology of cervical neoplasia, *J. Nutr.*, 123, 424, 1993.
2. Parker, S.L., Tong, T., Bolden, S., and Wingo, P.A., Cancer statistics 1997, *CA Cancer J. Clin.*, 47, 5, 1997.
3. Crum, C.P. and Nuovo, G.J., *Genital Papillomaviruses and Related Neoplasms*, Raven Press, New York, 1991, chap. 6.
4. Richart, R.M., Cervical intraepithelial neoplasia, in *Pathology Annual*, Sommers, S.C., Ed., Appleton-Century-Crofts, New York, 1973, 301.
5. Ostor, A.G., Natural history of cervical intraepithelial neoplasia: a critical review, *Int. J. Gynecol. Pathol.*, 12, 186, 1993.
6. Cotran, R.S., Kumar, V., and Robbins, S.L., *Robbins Pathologic Basis of Disease*, 5th ed., W.B. Saunders, Philadelphia, 1994, chap. 23.
7. Rotman, M., Madhu, J., and Boyce, J., Prognostic factors in cervical carcinoma: implications in staging and management, *Cancer*, 48, 560, 1981.

8. Taylor, R.R., Teneriello, M.G., Nash, J.D., Park, R.C., and Birrer, M.J., The molecular genetics of gyn malignancies, *Oncology*, 8, 63, 1994.

9. Baker, V., Oncogenes in gynecologic malignancy, *Curr. Opinion Obstet. Gynecol.*, 4, 75, 1992.

10. Riou, G., Barrois, M., Sheng, Z.M., Duvillard, P., and L'homme, C., Somatic deletions and mutations of c-Ha-*ras* gene in human cervical cancer cases, *Oncogene*, 3, 329, 1988.

11. Sagae, S., Kuzumaki, N., Hisada, T., Mugikura, Y., Kudo, R., and Hashimoto, M., *Ras* oncogene expression and prognosis of invasive squamous cell carcinoma of the uterine cervix, *Cancer*, 63, 1577, 1989.

12. Hayashi, Y., Toru, H., Iwasaka, T., Fukuda, K., Okuma, Y., Yokoyama, M., and Sugimori, H., Expression of *ras* oncogene product and EGF receptor in cervical squamous cell carcinomas and its relationship to lymph node involvement, *Gynecol. Oncol.*, 40, 147, 1991.

13. Riou, G., Bourhis, J., and Le, M.G., The c-*myc* protooncogene in invasive carcinomas of the uterine cervix, *Anticancer Res.*, 10, 1225, 1991.

14. Iwasaka, T., Yokoyama, M., Ochuchida, M., Matsuo, N., Hara, K., Fukuyama, K., Hachisuga, T., Fukuda, K., and Sugimori, H., Detection of human papilloma virus genome and analysis of expression of c-*myc* and Ha-*ras* oncogenes in invasive cervical carcinomas, *Gynecol. Oncol.*, 46, 298, 1992.

15. Bourhis, J., Le, M.G., Barrois, M., Gerbaulet, A., Jeannel, D., Duvillard, P., Le Dossal, V., Chassagne, D., and Riou, G., Prognostic value of c-*myc* protooncogene overexpression in early invasive carcinoma of the cervix, *J. Clin. Oncol.*, 8, 1789, 1990.

16. Ocadiz, R., Sauceda, R., Cruz, M., Graef, A.M., and Gariglio, P., High correlation between molecular alterations of the c-*myc* oncogene and carcinoma of the uterine cervix, *Cancer Res.*, 47, 4173, 1987.

17. Baker, V., Hatch, K.D., and Shingleton, H.M., Amplification of the c-*myc* protooncogene in cervical carcinoma, *J. Surg. Oncol.*, 39, 225, 1988.

18. Berchuck, A., Rodriquez, G., Kamel, A., Soper, J.T., Clarke-Pearson, D.L., and Bast, R.C., Jr., Expression of epidermal growth factor receptor and HER-2/neu in normal and neoplastic cervix, vulva, and vagina, *Obstet. Gynecol.*, 76, 381, 1990.

19. Pfeiffer, D., Stellwag, B., Pfeiffer, A., Borlinghaus, P., Meier, W., and Schneidel, P., Clinical implications of the epidermal growth factor receptor in the squamous cell carcinoma of the uterine cervix, *Gynecol. Oncol.*, 33, 146, 1989.

20. Hale, R.J., Buckley, C.H., Fox, H., and Williams, J., Prognostic value of c-erbB-2 expression in uterine cervical carcinoma, *J. Clin. Pathol.*, 45, 594, 1992.

21. Sreekantaiah, C., Bhargava, K., and Shetty, N.J., Chromosome 1 abnormalities in cervical carcinoma, *Cancer*, 62, 1317, 1988.

22. Chung, C.T., Huang, D.P., Lo, K.W., Chan, M.K., and Wong, F.W., Genetic lesions in the carcinogenesis of cervical cancer, *Anticancer Res.*, 12, 1485, 1992.

23. Kaelbling, M., Burk, R.D., Atkin, N.B., Johnson, A.B., and Klinger, H.P., Loss of heterozygosity on chromosome 17p and mutant *p53* in HPV negative cervical carcinomas, *Lancet*, 340, 140, 1992.

24. Russell, S.E., Lowry, W.S., Atkinson, R.J., and Hickey, I., Homozygosity of the short arm of chromosome 17 in cervical carcinoma, *Cancer Lett.*, 63, 243, 1992.

25. Fujita, M., Inoue, M., Tanizawa, O., Iwamoto, S., and Enomoto, T., Alterations of the *p53* gene in human primary cervical carcinoma with and without human papilloma virus infection, *Cancer Res.*, 52, 5323, 1992.

26. Crook, T., Wrede, D., Tidy, J.A., Mason, W.P., Evans, D.J., and Vousden, K.H., Clonal *p53* mutation in primary cervical cancer, *Lancet*, 339, 1070, 1992.

27. Tsuda, H. and Hirohashi, S., Frequent occurrence of *p53* gene mutations in uterine cancers at advanced clinical stage and with aggressive histological phenotypes, *Jpn. J. Cancer Res.*, 83, 1184, 1991.

28. Munger, K., Scheffner, M., Haibregtse, J.M., and Howley, P.M., Interactions of the HPV E6 and E7 oncoproteins with tumor suppressor gene products, *Cancer Surv.*, 12, 197, 1992.

29. Lynch, H.T., Lynch, J.F., Conway, T.A., and Bewtra, C., Genetics and gynecologic cancer, in *Principles and Practice of Gynecologic Oncology*, Hoslins, W.J., Perez, C.A., and Young, R.C., Eds., J.B. Lippincott, Philadelphia, 1992, 27.

30. Kullander, S., Hereditary factors in human cervical cancer, in *Cancer Genetics in Women*, Vol. II, Lynch, H.T. and Kullander, S., Eds., CRC Press, Boca Raton, FL, 1987, 113.

31. Shiffman, M.H., Brinton, L.A., Devesa, S.S., and Fraumeni, J.F., Jr., Cervical cancer, in *Cancer Epidemiology and Prevention*, 2nd ed., Schottenfeld, D. and Fraumeni, J.F., Jr., Eds., Oxford University Press, New York, 1996, 1096.

32. Bosch, F.X., Manos, M.M., Munoz, N., Sherman, M., Jansen, A.M., Peto, J., Schiffman, M.H., Morena, V., Kurman, R., and Shah, K.V., Prevalence of human papillomavirus in cervical cancer: a worldwide perspective, *J. Natl. Cancer Inst.*, 87, 796, 1995.

33. Burger, R.A., Monk, B.J., Kurosaki, T., Anton-Culver, H., Vasilev, S.A., Berman, M.L., and Wilczynski, S.P., Human papillomavirus type 18: association with poor prognosis in early stage cervical cancer, *J. Natl. Cancer Inst.*, 88, 1361, 1996.

34. Tattersall, M.H.N. and Rose, B.R., Prognostic factors for survival in cervical cancer—warts and all, *J. Natl. Cancer Inst.*, 88, 1331, 1996.

35. Bosch, F.X., Castellsague, X., Munoz, N., de Sanjose, S., Gjaffari, A.M., Gonzalez, L.C., Gile, M., Izarzugaza, I., Viladiu, P., Navarro, C., Vegara, A., Ascunce, N., Guerrero, E., and Shah, K.V., Male sexual behavior and human papillomavirus DNA: key risk factors for cervical cancer in Spain, *J. Natl. Cancer Inst.*, 88, 1060, 1996.

36. Munoz, N., Castellsague, X., Bosch, F.X., de Sanjose, S., Aristizabal, N., Ghaffari, A.M., and Shah, K.V., Difficulty in elucidating the male role in cervical cancer in Colombia, a high-risk area for the disease, *J. Natl. Cancer Inst.*, 88, 1068, 1996.

37. Noller, K.L., O'Brien, P.C., Melton, L.J. III, Offord, J.R., Richart, R.M., Robbay, S.J., and Kaufman, R.H., Coital risk factors for cervical cancer: sexual activity among white middle class women, *Am. J. Clin. Oncol.*, 10, 222, 1987.

38. Viaque, J. and Fenollar, J., The distribution of cervical cancer mortality in Spain (1981–1986): an ecological study, *Med. Clin.*, 104, 287, 1995.

39. Gardner, J.W., Schuman, K.L., Slattery, M.L., Sanborn, J.S., Abbott, T.M., and Overall, J.D., Jr., Is vaginal douching related to cervical carcinoma? *Am. J. Epidemiol.*, 133, 368, 1991.

40. Gram, I.T., Macaluso, M., Churchill, J., and Stalsberg, H., *Trichomonas vaginalis* (TV) and human papillomavirus infection and the incidence of cervical intraepithelial neoplasia (CIN) grade III, *Cancer Causes Control*, 3, 231, 1992.

41. Zhang, Z.F. and Begg, C.B., Is *Trichomonas vaginalis* a cause of cervical neoplasia? Results from a combined analysis of 24 studies, *Int. J. Epidemiol.*, 23, 682, 1994.

42. Zhang, Z.F., Graham, S., Yu, S.Z., Marshall, J., Zielezny, M., Chen, Y.X., Sun, M., Tang, S.L., Liao, C.S., Xu, J.L., and Yang, X.-Z., *Trichomonas vaginalis* and cervical cancer: a prospective study in China, *Ann. Epidemiol.*, 5, 325, 1995.

43. Phillips, A.N. and Smith, G.D., Cigarette smoking as a potential cause of cervical cancer: has confounding been controlled? *Int. J. Epidemiol.*, 23, 42, 1994.

44. WHO Collaborative Study of Neoplasia and Steroid Contraceptives: invasive squamous cell cervical carcinoma and combined oral contraceptive results from a multi-national study, *Int. J. Cancer*, 55, 228, 1993.

45. Bosch, F.X., Munoz, N., de Sanjose, S., Izarzugaza, I., Gili, M., Viladiu, P., Tormo, M.J., Moreo, P., Ascunce, N., Gonzalez, L.C., Tafur, L., Kaldor, J.M., Guerrero, E., Aristizabal, N., Santamaria, M., Alonso de Ruiz, P., and Shah, K., Risk factors for cervical cancer in Colombia and Spain, *Int. J. Cancer*, 52, 750, 1992.

46. Eluf-Neto, J., Booth, M., Munoz, N., Bosch, F.X., Meijer, C.J., and Walboomers, J.M., Human papillomavirus and invasive cancer in Brazil, *Br. J. Cancer*, 69, 114, 1994.

47. Wylie-Rosett, J.A., Romney, S.L., Slagle, N.S., Wassertheil-Smoller, S., Miller, G.L., Palan, P.R., Lucido, D.J., and Duttagupta, C., Influence of vitamin A on cervical dysplasia and carcinoma *in situ*, *Nutr. Cancer*, 6, 49, 1984.

48. Liu, T., Soong, S.-J., Wilson, N.P., Craig, C.B., Cole, P., Macaluso, M., and Butterworth, C.E., Jr., A case control study of nutritional factors and cervical dysplasia, *Cancer Epidemiol. Biomarkers Prev.*, 2, 525, 1993.

49. La Vecchia, C., Decarli, A., Fasoli, M., Parazzini, F., Franceschi, S., Gentile, A., and Negri, E., Dietary vitamin A and the risk of intraepithelial and invasive cervical neoplasia, *Gynecol. Oncol.*, 30, 187, 1988.

50. Brock, K.E., Berry, G., Mock, P.A., MacLennan, R., Truswell, A.S., and Brinton, L.A., Nutrients in diet and plasma and risk of *in situ* cervical cancer, *J. Natl. Cancer Inst.*, 80, 580, 1988.

51. Marshall, J.R., Graham, S., Byers, T., Swanson, M., and Brasure, J., Diet and smoking in the epidemiology of cancer of the cervix, *J. Natl. Cancer Inst.*, 70, 847, 1983.

52. Verreault, R., Chu, J., Mandelson, M., and Shy, K., A case-control study of diet and invasive cervical cancer, *Int. J. Cancer*, 43, 1050, 1989.

53. Herrero, R., Potischman, N., Brinton, L.A., Reeves, W.C., Brenes, M.M., Tenorio, F., deBritton, R.C., and Gaitan, E., A case-control study of nutrient status and invasive cervical cancer. I. Dietary indicators, *Am. J. Epidemiol.*, 134, 1335, 1991.

54. Van Eenwyk, J., Davis, F.G., and Bowen, P.E., Dietary and serum carotenoids and cervical intraepithelial neoplasia, *Int. J. Cancer*, 48, 34, 1991.

55. Ziegler, R.G., Jones, C.J., Brinton, L.A., Norman, S.A., Mallin, K., Levine, R.S., Lehman, H.F., Hamman, R.F., Trumble, A.C., Rosenthal, J.F., and Hoover, R.N.,

Diet and the risk of *in situ* cervical cancer among white women in the United States, *Cancer Causes Control*, 2, 17, 1991.

56. Slattery, M.L., Abbott, T.M., Overall, J.C., Robison, L.M., French, T.K., Jolles, C., Gardner, J.W., and West, D.W., Dietary vitamins A, C, and E and selenium as risk factors for cervical cancer, *Epidemiology*, 1, 8, 1990.

57. Ziegler, R.G., Brinton, L.A., Hamman, R.F., Lehman, H.F., Levine, R.S., Mallin, K., Norman, S.A., Rosenthal, J.F., Trumble, A.C., and Hoover, R.N., Diet and the risk of invasive cervical cancer among white women in the United States, *Am. J. Epidemiol.*, 132, 432, 1990.

58. de Vet, H.C., Knipschild, P.G., Grol, M.E.C., Schouten, H.J.A., and Sturmans, F., The role of beta-carotene and other dietary factors in the etiology of cervical dysplasia: results of a case-control study, *Int. J. Epidemiol.*, 20, 603, 1991.

59. Harris, R.W.C., Forman, D., Doll, R., Vessey, M.P., and Wald, N.J., Cancer of the cervix uteri and vitamin A, *Br. J. Cancer*, 53, 653, 1986.

60. Lambert, B., Brisson, G., and Bielman, P., Plasma vitamin A and precancerous lesions of cervix uteri: a preliminary report, *Gynecol. Oncol.*, 11, 136, 1981.

61. Heinonen, P.K., Kuoppala, T., Koskinen, T., and Punnonen, R., Serum vitamins A and E and carotene in patients with gynecologic cancer, *Arch. Gynecol. Obstet.*, 241, 151, 1987.

62. Potischman, N., Hoover, R.N., Brinton, L.A., Swanson, C.A., Herrero, R., Tenorio, F., deBritton, R.C., Gaitan, E., and Reeves, W.C., The relations between cervical cancer and serological markers of nutritional status, *Nutr. Cancer*, 21, 193, 1994.

63. Manetta, A., Schubbert, T., Chapman, J., Schell, M.J., Peng, Y.-M., Liao, S.Y., and Meyskens, F.J., Jr., β-Carotene treatment of cervical intraepithelial neoplasia: a phase II study, *Cancer Epidemiol. Biomarkers Prev.*, 5, 929, 1996.

64. Orr, J.W., Wilson, K., Bodiford, C., Cornwell, A., Soong, S.J., Honea, K.L., Hatch, K.D., and Singleton, H.M., Nutritional status of patients with untreated cervical cancer. II. Vitamin assessment, *Am. J. Obstet. Gynecol.*, 151, 632, 1985.

65. Romney, S.L., Duttagupta, C., Basu, J., Palan, P.R., Karp, S., Slagle, N.S., Dwyer, A., Wassertheil-Smoller, S., and Wylie-Rosett, J., Plasma vitamin C and uterine cervical dyaplasia, *Am. J. Obstet. Gynecol.*, 151, 976, 1985.

66. Basu, J., Palan, P.R., Vermund, S.H., Goldberg, G.L., Burk, R.D., and Romney, S.L., Plasma ascorbic acid and beta-carotene levels in women evaluated for HPV infection, smoking, and cervix dysplasia, *Cancer Detect. Prev.*, 15, 165, 1991.

67. Food and Nutrition Board, National Research Council, *Recommended Dietary Allowances*, 10th ed., National Academy Press, Washington, D.C., 1989.

68. Palan, P.R., Mikhail, M.S., Basu, J., and Romney, S.L., Plasma levels of antioxidant beta-carotene and alpha-tocopherol in uterine cervix dysplasias and cancer, *Nutr. Cancer*, 15, 13, 1991.

69. Cuzick, J., DeStavola, B.L., Russell, M.J., and Thomas, B.S., Vitamin A, vitamin E and the risk of cervical intraepithelial neoplasia, *Br. J. Cancer*, 62, 651, 1990.

70. Knekt, P., Serum vitamin E levels and risk of female cancers, *Int. J. Epidemiol.*, 17, 281, 1988.

71. Peritz, E., Ramcharan, S., Frank, J., Brown, W.L., Huang, S., and Ray, R., The incidence of cervical cancer and duration of oral contraceptive use, *Am. J. Epidemiol.*, 106, 462, 1977.

72. Stern, E., Steroid contraceptive use and cervical dysplasia: increased risk of progression, *Science*, 196, 1460, 1977.

73. Swan, S.H. and Brown, W.L., Oral contraceptive use, sexual activity and cervical carcinoma, *Am. J. Obstet. Gynecol.*, 139, 52, 1981.

74. Vessey, M.P., Lawless, M., McPherson, Y., and Yeates, D., Neoplasia of the cervix uteri and contraception: a possible adverse effect of the pill, *Lancet*, 2, 930, 1983.

75. Whitehead, N., Reyner, F., and Lindenbaum, J., Megaloblastic changes in the cervical epithelium: association with oral contraceptive therapy and reversal with folic acid, *J. Am. Med. Assoc.*, 226, 1421, 1973.

76. Butterworth, C.E., Jr., Hatch, K.D., Gore, H., Mueller, H., and Krumdieck, C.L., Improvement in cervical dysplasia associated with folic acid therapy in users of oral contraceptives, *Am. J. Clin. Nutr.*, 35, 73, 1982.

77. Butterworth, C.E., Jr., Hatch, K.D., Soong, S.-J., Cole, P., Tamura, T., Sauberlich, H.E., Borst, M., Macaluso, M., and Baker, V., Oral folic acid supplementation for cervical dysplasia: a clinical intervention trial, *Am. J. Obstet. Gynecol.*, 166, 803, 1992.

78. Butterworth, C.E., Jr., Folic acid deficiency and cervical dysplasia, in *Vitamins and Cancer Prevention*, Bray, G.H. and Ryan, D.H., Eds., Louisiana State University Press, Baton Rouge, 1993, 196.

79. Borst, M., Butterworth, C.E., Jr., Baker, V., Kuykendall, K., Gore, H., Soong, S., and Hatch, K.D., Human papillomavirus screening for women with atypical Papanicolaou smears, *J. Reprod. Med.*, 36, 95, 1991.

80. Popescu, N.C., Amspaugh, S.C., and Di Paolo, J.A., Human papillomavirus type 18 DNA is integrated at a single chromosome site in cervical carcinoma cell line, *J. Virol.*, 61, 1682, 1987.

81. Van Eenwyk, J., Davis, F.G., and Colman, N., Folate, vitamin C, and cervical intraepithelial neoplasia, *Cancer Epidemiol. Biomarkers Prev.*, 1, 119, 1992.

82. McPherson, R.S., Nutritional factors and the risk of cervical dysplasia, *Am. J. Epidemiol.*, 130, 830, 1989.

83. Butterworth, C.E., Hatch, K.D., Macaluso, M., Cole, P., Sauberlich, H.E., Soong, S.-J., Borst, M., and Baker, V.V., Folate deficiency and cervical dysplasia, *J. Am. Med. Assoc.*, 267, 528, 1992.

84. Potischman, N., Brinton, L.A., Laiming, V.A., Reeves, W.C., Brenes, M.M., Herrero, R., Tenorio, F., deBritton, R.C., and Gaitan, E., A case-control study of serum folate levels and invasive cervical cancer, *Cancer Res.*, 51, 47785, 1991.

85. Schneider, A., Morabia, A., Papendick, U., and Kirchmayr, R., Pork intake and human papillomavirus-related disease, *Nutr. Cancer*, 13, 209, 1990.

86. Potischman, N. and Brinton, L.A., Nutritional epidemiology of cervical cancer, *Cancer Causes Control*, 7, 113, 1996.

CHAPTER 4

NUTRITION AND CANCER OF THE OVARY

CONTENTS

I. GENERAL PATHOLOGY AND STATISTICS

A. Frequency of Occurrence

Ovarian cancer accounts for about 4% of all newly diagnosed cancers in women and 5% of all cancer-related deaths.[1] There are a number of tumor types in the ovary, as shown in Table 4.1. The most common are serous (40%) followed by endometrioid carcinomas (20%).[2]

Table 4.1   Certain Frequency Data for Major Ovarian Tumors

Type	Percentage of Malignant Ovarian Tumors	Percentage That Are Bilateral
Serous	40	
Benign (60%)		25
Borderline (15%)		30
Malignant (25%)		65
Mucinous	10	
Benign (80%)		5
Borderline (10%)		10
Malignant (10%)		20
Endometrioid carcinoma	20	40
Undifferentiated carcinoma	10	—
Clear cell carcinoma	6	40
Granulosa cell tumor	5	5
Teratoma		15
Benign (96%)		
Malignant (4%)	1	Rare
Metastatic	5	>50
Others	3	—

From Cotran, R.S., Kumar, V., and Robbins, S.L., *Robbins Pathologic Basis of Disease*, 5th ed., W.B. Saunders, Philadelphia, 1994, 1066. With permission.

B. Histologic Types

Both serous and mucinous tumors of the ovary can be divided into cystadenoma, tumor of low malignant potential, and cystadenocarcinoma.[3] Serous cystadenoma histologically demonstrates a single layer of tall columnar ciliated cells or can be cuboidal due to presence of cyst contents. They can be unilocular or multilocular grossly. There are few or no papillary excrescences and no solid areas; 20% are bilateral. It is a benign tumor which is cured by excision.

Serous tumor of low malignant potential demonstrates histologically complex papillary projections (tufts) and stratification of the epithelium with atypia and occasional mitosis. There tends to be no stromal invasion, and 45% are bilateral. The 5-year survival when confined to the ovary is 100%, but is 90% with peritoneal involvement (10-year survival is 75%).

Serous cystadenocarcinoma accounts for approximately 40% of all ovarian cancers and is the most common malignant ovarian tumor. Histologically, it shows invasion of the stroma, often by poorly differentiated bizarre cells, but most have a papillary architecture with associated psammoma bodies.[4] Greater than 60% are bilateral. The 5-year survival when the tumor is confined to the ovary is 70%, but when involving the peritoneum is only 25%.

Mucinous cystadenoma usually presents as multilocular cysts grossly lined by a single layer of tall mucinous ("endocervical"-like cells) microscopically.

Only approximately 5% are bilateral. This is a benign tumor that is cured by excision. Mucinous tumor of low malignant potential histologically shows papillary growth or stratification with up to four cells in depth with nuclear atypia and mitosis. The 10-year survival is 95%. Mucinous cystadenocarcinoma microscopically shows a more solid growth pattern with varied cellular atypia, stratification, loss of glandular architecture, and necrosis. Stromal invasion can be difficult to define in mucinous tumors. This tumor accounts for about 10% of all ovarian carcinomas. With peritoneal seeding, it may produce pseudomyxoma peritonei. The overall 10-year survival is about 65%.[5]

Endometrioid carcinoma is a malignant tumor with glands resembling endometrial carcinoma. About 15–30% are accompanied by carcinoma of the endometrium, and 15% coexist with endometriosis. The overall 5-year survival is about 40–50%.[6] Clear cell adenocarcinoma is composed of large cells with abundant clear cytoplasm, and it frequently occurs along with endometrial carcinoma. It may be predominantly solid or cystic grossly, and it usually presents peri- or postmenopausally. When confined to the ovary, the overall 5-year survival is about 50%; with spread, most patients survive less than 5 years.[7]

Brenner tumors histologically show nests of cells resembling transitional epithelium within a dense fibrous stroma. The cells frequently have nuclear grooves.[8] The majority of Brenner tumors are benign, with rare reports of borderline or malignant counterparts. Transitional cell carcinoma is histologically similar to epithelial tumors of the urinary bladder with an absence of Brenner tumor component. This carcinoma is associated with an especially good response to chemotherapy.

Mature teratomas are mostly cystic (dermoid cysts) containing hair, sebaceous material, teeth, and other mature tissues. Many are incidental findings in young women.[9] About 1% of teratomas undergo malignant transformation in one or more of the components. Most often squamous cell carcinoma develops. Immature malignant teratomas are different from mature teratomas in that the tissue components resemble that of an embryo or fetus rather than an adult. They are predominantly solid tumors with areas of necrosis and hemorrhage, and the histologic grade is based on the immature neuroepithelial component. Most recurrences develop within the first 2 years.[10] Monodermal teratomas most commonly are struma ovarii composed entirely of mature thyroid tissue, which may cause hyperthyroidism, and ovarian carcinoid, which may cause carcinoid syndrome. In rare cases, strumal carcinoid can occur, which is a combination of struma ovarii and carcinoid tumor in the same ovary.[10]

Dysgerminoma histologically shows sheets and nests of large vesicular cells with clear cytoplasm with associated lymphocytes. It is best thought of as the ovarian counterpart of the seminoma in the testis. Most occur in young adults in their second and third decades. They are usually unilateral and are extremely radiosensitive. The 5-year survival is 70–90%.[11] Endodermal sinus tumor (yolk sac tumor) is an embryonal carcinoma with differentiation toward yolk sac structures (Schiller-Duval body). The tumor produces alpha-fetoprotein and alpha-1 antitrypsin, which may be helpful in diagnosis and as a marker of recurrence. This is a rapidly growing aggressive tumor. It was once uniformly fatal, but chemotherapy has improved the prognosis.[12]

Choriocarcinoma is a malignant germ cell tumor with differentiation toward placental tissue, with a combination of both cytotrophoblasts and syncytiotrophoblasts. Histologically, it produces human chorionic gonadotropin. A pure choriocarcinoma is extremely rare and is usually a component of a mixed germ cell tumor. Unlike placental choriocarcinoma, these tumors are generally unresponsive to chemotherapy and carry a very poor prognosis, having generally widely metastasized through the bloodstream prior to diagnosis.[12]

Granulosa-theca cell tumors are estrogen-secreting and can take on many histological variations but characteristically have Call-Exner bodies present. They are of low-grade malignancy and carry a good prognosis.[13] Thecoma-fibromas arise from either fibroblasts (fibromas) or plump spindle cells with liquid droplets (thecomas) or combinations of both cell types. These tumors may cause ascites in about 40% of cases. The ascites may uncommonly be in association with hydrothorax (Meig's syndrome).[14]

Sertoli-Leydig cell tumors (androblastoma) usually produce androgenic hormones presenting with features of virilization. These tumors recapitulate the cells of the testis at various stages of development. The increase of recurrence or metastasis by Sertoli-Leydig cell tumors is less than 5%.[15] Gonadoblastoma is a mixed neoplasm consisting of germ cells and a sex cord–stromal component. Nests of a mixture of cells resembling immature Sertoli and granulosa cells are seen microscopically.[16] It is usually associated with gonadal dysgenesis, and a coexistent dysgerminoma occurs in 50% of cases. Prognosis is excellent with complete tumor excision. With regard to metastatic tumors, the Krukenberg tumor refers to bilateral ovarian metastases of mucin-producing signet ring cancer cells, usually of gastric origin.[17] Staging of ovarian cancers is presented in Table 4.2.[18]

II. POPULATION GENETICS AND MARKERS FOR RISK

A. Family History

Family history has been studied for a number of years as a risk factor for ovarian cancer. Kerber and Slattery[19] examined the impact of family history on ovarian cancer risk using the Utah Population Database, which is a genealogy of about one million people linked to cancer incidence data from the Utah Cancer Registry. Using this database, they concluded that family histories of ovarian, uterine, breast, and pancreatic cancer were significantly associated with increased risk of ovarian cancer. The risk of ovarian cancer was substan-

TABLE 4.2 International Federation of Gynecology and Obstetrics (FIGO) Stage Grouping for Primary Carcinoma of the Ovary (1987)

Stage	Description
Stage I	Growth limited to the ovaries
Stage IA	Growth limited to one ovary, no ascites; no tumor on the external surfaces, capsules intact
Stage IB	Growth limited to both ovaries, no ascites; no tumor on the external surfaces, capsules intact
Stage IC	Tumor stage IA or IB but with tumor on the surface of one or both ovaries, with capsule ruptured, with ascites present containing malignant cells, or with positive peritoneal washings
Stage II	Growth involving one or both ovaries with pelvic extension
Stage IIA	Extension or metastases to the uterus or tubes
Stage IIB	Growth involving one or both ovaries with pelvic extension
Stage IIC	Tumor either stage IIA or IIB but with tumor on the surface of one or both ovaries, with capsules ruptured, with ascites present containing malignant cells, or with positive peritoneal washings
Stage III	Tumor involving one or both ovaries with peritoneal implants outside the pelvis or positive retroperitoneal or inguinal nodes, superficial liver metastases equal stage III; tumor limited to the true pelvis but with histologically verified malignant extension to small bowel or omentum
Stage IIIA	Tumor grossly limited to the true pelvis with negative nodes but with histologically confirmed microscopic seeding of abdominal peritoneal surfaces
Stage IIIB	Tumor of one or both ovaries with histologically confirmed implants of abdominal peritoneal surfaces, none exceeding 2 cm in diameter; nodes negative
Stage IIIC	Abdominal implants >2 cm in diameter, or positive retroperitoneal or inguinal nodes
Stage IV	Growth involving one or both ovaries with distant metastasis; if pleural effusion is present, there must be positive cytologic test results to allot a case to stage IV; parenchymal liver metastasis equals stage IV

From DeVita, V.T., Hellman, S., and Rosenberg, S.A., *Cancer: Principles and Practice of Oncology*, 5th ed., Lippincott-Raven Publishers, Philadelphia, 1997, chap. 35. With permission.

tially increased among women with family histories not only of ovarian cancer, but also uterine, pancreatic, and to a lesser extent breast cancer. High parity does not appear to be protective in women with a family history of ovarian cancer.[19]

In terms of genetics and women's cancer in general, according to Narod,[20] it is important to distinguish between hereditary and familial cancers. The term "familial cancer" is mostly used by epidemiologists to define a subgroup of cancer patients with a positive family history of breast or ovarian cancer, and it may be hereditary or may simply be a chance occurrence.[20] There are five types of hereditary cancer: (1) site-specific breast cancer, (2) site-specific ovarian cancer, (3) breast/ovarian cancer syndrome, (4) Li-Fraumeni syndrome, and (5) hereditary nonpolyposis colon cancer (HNPCC).[20] The most important criterion in making a diagnosis of hereditary ovarian cancer is the total number of family members affected with the cancer. The Breast Cancer Linkage Consortium has determined that three cases of ovarian cancer in first-degree relatives is considered hereditary site-specific cancer.[20]

B. *BRCA1* and *BRCA2*

In terms of genetic susceptibility to cancer of the ovary, it has been found that the same gene on human chromosome 17q12-q21 predisposes to both cancer of the breast and of the ovary. This gene, *BRCA1*, linked to the D17S74 locus, was discovered in 1990 by Dr. Mary-Claire King and colleagues, and shortly thereafter, linkage was also established for three of five families with breast-ovarian cancer (see Narod[20] for review). The estimated frequency of carriers of *BRCA1* mutations is 1 in 500, and its penetrance in the population varies according to age. The estimated proportion of breast cancer due to mutations in *BRCA1* ranges from 28% for those cases less than 30 years of age to less than 1% for those over 70. The cumulative risk for ovarian cancer is 48% up to age 70 and 85% for breast cancer.[20] In 1994, a second breast cancer susceptibility gene was discovered by Wooster et al.,[21] which localized to chromosome 13q12-13. This gene was designated *BRCA2*, not *RB1*, although it occurs in the same region of 13q.[22] *BRCA2* is purported to be another tumor suppressor gene with demonstrated loss of heterozygosity in ovarian cancer cases. Its loss confers a high risk of early-onset breast cancer in females, but it confers a much lower ovarian cancer risk than *BRCA1*. Studies are currently under way to estimate the penetrance of the *BRCA2* gene and the possibility that it may be causing other cancers.[22]

Recent studies on the frequency of the above gene mutations have focused on Jewish women with ovarian cancer. Since the first breast/ovarian cancer susceptibility gene, *BRCA1,* was cloned, more than 38 distinct germline mutations have been found among individuals with the hereditary syndrome.[23] A particular mutation, *185delAG,* has been described in at least ten Jewish families of Ashkenazi origin and has been found recently to occur with a prevalence of 0.9% in Jewish individuals.[23] It has subsequently been estimated that this particular mutation accounts for 16% of breast cancers and 39% of the ovarian cancers occurring in Ashkenazi women before 50 years of age. Muto et al.[23] reported that 19% of Jewish patients were carriers for this mutation compared to non-Jewish controls and estimated the relative risk associated with a *185delAG* mutation to be 12.0. For ovarian cancer diagnosed prior to 50 years, 37.5% carried the mutation.[23] In further analysis of mutations in the *BRCA2* gene, Berman et al.[24] used allele-specific PCR to screen for the *617delT* mutation in Jewish and non-Jewish women who had cancer and also a strong family history of breast/ovarian cancer. They found that this particular mutation is present within both the Jewish Ashkenazi and non-Jewish populations, and there may be several independent origins for the mutation. The authors are hopeful that their results will make it possible to develop rapid and effective screening methods for determining *BRCA2* carrier status in cancer patients.[24] However, few somatic *BRCA1* mutations have been found in sporadic ovarian tumors and none in sporadic breast tumors.[25] Although loss of heterozygosity studies have shown that both *BRCA1* and *BRCA2* are frequently deleted in sporadic breast and ovarian cancer, somatic mutations of *BRCA2* have also been found to be infrequent in sporadic ovarian cancer.[25]

C. Oncogenes

Other genes examined for relevance to ovarian cancer are *HRAS1* and *TP53*.[20] A meta-analysis of the occurrence of polymorphisms in the *HRAS1* gene has shown them to be associated with a 1.93 times increased risk of breast cancer, but no information is available for the association between this locus and ovarian cancer.[20,22] Hereditary nonpolyposis colon cancer genes can predispose individuals to cancers at other sites besides the colon, including the ovaries. Watson and Lynch[26] estimated the risk of ovarian cancer in members of 23 *HNPCC* kindreds to be approximately four times greater than that of the general population. In 1990, Malkin et al.[27] reported that five of five Li-Fraumeni syndrome families had germline mutations of the *p53* gene, although it has been thought that these mutations do not account for any breast or ovarian cancer outside of the Li-Fraumeni syndrome.[22] In summary, Ford and Easton[22] have stated that "it is now clear that most breast-ovarian families are caused by *BRCA1* and some, possibly all, of the remainder are due to *BRCA2*." But the caveat is that even with the high penetrance of genes such as *BRCA1* and *BRCA2*, and to a lesser extent with *TP53* and *HNPCC*, these are still likely to account for less than 10% of all breast/ovarian cancer cases in the population.[22]

D. Biomarkers for Risk

Markers for risk of ovarian cancer that would aid in screening those individuals with a substantially increased genetic risk are not currently available. More advances have been made in the area of prognostic indicators than in the area of screening or premalignant biomarkers of risk. One such marker is the prognostic significance of the *p53* tumor suppressor gene product. Immunostaining of paraffin-embedded specimens for *p53* expression in stage I ovarian cancer patients was reported,[28] and *p53* expression was associated with grade 3 to 4 disease. Although abnormalities of *p53* expression were associated with decreased survival in a univariate analysis, this biomarker did not retain its independence in a multivariate analysis and should be studied in a larger cohort of stage I patients.[28] The circulating tumor marker CA-125 has been used to follow women with epithelial ovarian cancers and has been employed in differentiating benign from malignant tumors.[29] It is also being tested in various programs for its role in the early detection of cancer of the ovary, where 5-year survival rates for stage I and II disease are 90 and 70%, respectively. However, there is a high false positivity rate associated with CA-125, even when followed by ultrasound examination.[29] Unfortunately, although developments in the molecular genetics of ovarian cancer may eventually prove useful with family histories of this disease, it is thought that these represent only about 3% of women who develop epithelial ovarian cancer.[29]

III. GENERAL EPIDEMIOLOGY OF OVARIAN CANCER

A. Oral Contraceptive Use

Similar to endometrial cancer, ovarian cancer is more common in the United States and other Western countries than in Asia and is also correlated with cancers of the breast, colon, and endometrium. Ovarian cancer also tends to occur more frequently in women in the higher socioeconomic groups, which may point to some dietary etiologic factors that will be discussed in the following sections. There have been a number of hormone-related factors which have been examined in recent years, especially the use of oral contraceptives.[30–35] A WHO Collaborative Study of Neoplasia and Steroid Hormones in 1989 investigated the relationship between the use of combined oral contraceptives and the risk of epithelial ovarian cancer in a hospital-based case-control study. It found that the relative risk for cancer decreased with increasing duration of oral contraceptive use and increasing time since cessation of use. The reduced risk seen with oral contraceptive use was present in parous women, but was more pronounced in nulliparous women (relative risk [RR] = 0.16). The negative association seen was similar for developing as well as developed countries. A more recent study by Gross et al.[35] followed up on the WHO study to attempt to determine what mechanisms might account for the negative correlation with even very short-term use of oral contraceptives. The authors compared cases with controls for factors such as age, parity, family history of ovarian cancer, estrogen dose, history of sterilization, and latency defined as time interval from first use of oral contraceptives. Their analyses suggested that the short-term (3–6 months) use of oral contraceptives has little to no effect on reduction in risk of epithelial ovarian cancer and that cessation of use due to side effects shortly after begun may indicate the presence of factors that are protective against the disease but have nothing to do with oral contraceptive use per se.[35]

B. Reproductive Function

There have also been other hypotheses related to women's reproductive function that have been investigated for a relationship to development of ovarian cancer. One such study examined the relationship between tubal sterilization, hysterectomy, and the subsequent occurrence of epithelial ovarian cancer in women aged 20–54 years in eight population-based cancer registries in the

United States and who were diagnosed during 1980–82.[36] Controls were obtained from randomly selected female residents of the same geographic areas. Women who had had tubal sterilization (RR = 0.69), hysterectomy only (RR = 0.55), or hysterectomy with oophorectomy (RR = 0.60) had lower risks of subsequently developing ovarian cancer. The authors[36] conclude that these findings may be explained by the fact that pelvic surgery is often accompanied by screening for occult ovarian pathology, although they could not rule out hormonal or other factors. Mori et al.[37] in Japan found that ovarian cancer risk was increased in single women and in women with a family history of the disease and that risk was decreased by live birth, induced abortion, or tubal ligation. More recent studies[38] into characteristics relating to ovarian cancer risk have supported the association of family history with increased risk of the disease and that increased numbers of pregnancies, increasing length of oral contraceptive use, and increasing duration of lactation are protective. A history of breast or endometrial cancer appears to be associated with a small elevation in risk as well. Continued interest in the impact of lactation on ovarian cancer risk showed discordant results. Rosenblatt and Thomas[39] reported a nonsignificant effect on risk reduction with short-term lactation and no further reduction in risk with long-term lactation. Months of pregnancy was a greater reducer of risk than months of lactation, and the authors speculate that this may be due to the more effective suppression of ovarian function with pregnancy than with lactation.

Infertility treatments are another variable examined for their relationship to risk for cancers of the ovary.[38] Three studies were analyzed for the role of infertility treatments and found them to be associated with increased risk (RR = 2.8), especially in nulligravid women. However, these results have been challenged by de Mouzon et al.,[40] who said that bias cannot be ruled out and that a large epidemiology study should be undertaken to fully investigate this association. In contrast, there has also been a report demonstrating a protective effect of pregnancy and breast-feeding on risk for ovarian cancer.[41] Logistic regression analysis demonstrated a strong trend in decreased risk of epithelial ovarian cancer with increased cumulative months of pregnancy. A marked reduction in risk was also seen for ever having breast-fed and the use of oral contraceptives, although the greatest effects were seen for cumulative months of pregnancy.[41]

Expanding investigations into the use of steroid hormones and epithelial ovarian cancer, another study from the WHO Collaborative Study of Neoplasia and Steroid Contraceptives conducted in 1991[42] examined the use of depomedroxyprogesterone (DMPA) in a hospital-based case-control study in Mexico and Thailand. The authors concluded[42] that no consistent patterns of increased or decreased risk were seen and that the risk of epithelial ovarian cancer is not altered by the use of DMPA.

Previous epidemiologic studies have focused mostly on white women, since they have a higher incidence of ovarian cancer than black women. One study has analyzed in a case-control study characteristics of risk in U.S. black women for epithelial ovarian cancer.[43] Characteristics evaluated were pregnancy, oral contraceptive use, and breast-feeding. Decreased rates of cancer were found with parity of four or more (odds ratio [OR] = 0.53), breast-feeding for 6 months or more (OR = 0.85), and the use of oral contraceptives for 6 years or longer (OR = 0.62). The authors concluded that although a greater proportion of black (48%) than white (27%) women had greater than four pregnancies and were more likely to breast-feed, and more white than black women reported oral contraceptive use, differences in genetic susceptibility must explain most of the differences in rates of ovarian cancer between black and white women.[43]

Finally, in terms of nonhormonally related etiologic factors in cancer of the ovary, Harlow and Hartge[44] reviewed the evidence for talc as a potential ovarian carcinogen. They concluded that the range of relative risks was 1.0–1.8 and that causality may be plausible, but that additional studies are warranted, especially pathology documentation of talc migration into ovarian tissue.

IV. DIETARY FAT, BODY WEIGHT, AND FAT DISTRIBUTION

A. Obesity, Body Mass, and Fat Distribution

A number of studies have been performed in an attempt to relate nutritional factors, obesity, and body fat distribution to the risk for epithelial ovarian cancer. However, a couple of early epidemiological studies showed no association between cancer cases and obesity or height/weight. In one case-control study in 1979, Annegers et al.[45] observed that obesity was not a risk factor for ovarian cancer, and in one other study the authors found no effect of height or weight.[46] Adipose tissue distribution in women participants in a longitudinal study in Göteborg, Sweden, was analyzed for association with endometrial or ovarian carcinoma.[47] Measurements of generalized obesity as body weight or body mass index or peripherally localized adipose tissue as determined by triceps skinfold measurements showed no associations with either ovarian or endometrial cancers.[47] Although a positive association was seen with occurrence and incidence data for endometrial and ovarian cancer, the association of centrally located adipose tissue (waist circumference) to endometrial and ovarian carcinoma did not hold up in a multivariate analysis when generalized obesity was also a factor.[47] The conclusions from the Committee on Diet and Health of the National Research Council in 1989[48] have previously determined that most studies of weight and height did not find an association with ovarian cancer risk, and these seem to have been upheld since then. However, two recent studies have examined variations on the theme of body weight and have reported some interesting conclusions. Barker et al.[49] studied women in the United Kingdom with ovarian cancer and the amount of weight gain during infancy. They found that those who died from cancer of the ovary had had a higher rate of weight gain in infancy, although their mean birth weight was the same as that of other women. The authors concluded that ovarian cancer may be linked to altered patterns of gonadotropin release established in utero when the fetal hypothalamus is imprinted.[49] Another study of lifelong physical activity and cancer risk was examined among female teachers in Finland.[50] The study found that the standardized incidence ratios for all cancers in those teachers was essentially the same, with both groups having elevated cancers of the breast, endometrium, ovary, and colon, so that no effect of exercise was evident.

B. Specific Dietary Factors

Specific dietary variables have been studied since the early 1980s when Cramer et al.[51] found that women with ovarian cancer consumed significantly greater amounts of animal fat and considerably less vegetable fat than did controls (Table 4.3). However, in contrast, Byers et al.[52] found no such association. Rose et al.[53] compared the mortality rates for cancers of the breast, prostate, ovary, and colon in 26–30 countries to the average food availability data published by the United Nations. Although this type of ecological study can only be a gross association, they found that the excess mortality from breast and ovarian cancer in Israel was related to the national animal fat consumption. They postulated[53] that the observed positive correlations between four cancer sites and caloric intake from animal sources, along with negative associations with consumption of fat from vegetable sources, indicated that animal fat and

Table 4.3   Studies of Dietary Factors and Ovarian Cancer Risk

Nutrient	Type of Study	Association with Risk	Reference
Animal fat	Case-control	Increased	Cramer et al.[51]
	Case-control	No association	Byers et al.[52]
	Ecological	Excess mortality	Rose et al.[53]
	Case-control	Increased, OR = 1.8	Shu et al.[55]
Vegetables	Ecological	Inverse	Rose et al.[53]
Calories, fat, protein, fiber, vitamins A and C	Case-control	No association	Slattery et al.[54]
Beta-carotene	Case-control	Inverse, OR = 0.5	Slattery et al.[54]
Fat-rich foods	Ecological	Increased death rates	Kato et al.[56]
Fat-containing foods	Mortality trends	Increased cancer	Serra-Majem et al.[61]
Meat	Case-control	Attributable risk = 19.2%	Mori and Miyake[57]
	Case-control	Increased, RR = 1.6	La Vecchia et al.[58]
All dietary factors	Case-control	No association	Tzonou et al.[60]
Coffee	Case-control	Increased	La Vecchia et al.[63]
			Trichopoulos et al.[64]
	Case-control	No association	Byers et al.[52]
Lactose	Case-control	Decreased, OR = 0.3	Harlow et al.[66]
	Case-control	No association	Engle et al.[68]
			Risch et al.[69]
Galactose	Case-control	Increased	Cramer[67]
Alcohol	Case-control	Increased, RR = 1.3	La Vecchia et al.[70]

not energy is the major dietary influence on risk for these four cancers. Slattery et al.[54] reported on nutrient intake and ovarian cancer, looking specifically at calories, fat, protein, fiber, and vitamins A and C, and found that their intake did not appreciably alter the risk for ovarian cancer. However, a high intake of beta-carotene appeared to confer some protection, with an OR of 0.5.[54] Shu et al.[55] also reported that when they analyzed dietary data from a case-control study, a significant dose–response relationship was found between the intake of fat from animal sources and the risk of ovarian cancer (OR = 1.8 for upper quartile). Total vegetable intake was found to be somewhat protective. In a Japanese study of the relationship between the Westernization of dietary habits and mortality from breast and ovarian cancers, the authors[56] reported that an increased consumption of Western-style fat-rich foods such as butter and margarine, cheese, bread, ham, and sausage among Japanese women might be associated with recent increases in age-adjusted death rates for both breast and ovarian cancers. Another Japanese case-control study of reproductive, genetic, and dietary risk factors for ovarian cancer[37] found that there was a significant positive association with daily fish consumption and a marginally negative association with daily milk consumption. The same authors[57] examined dietary and other risk factors for ovarian cancer among elderly women and reported that daily meat consumption was significantly associated with the occurrence of ovarian cancer, with an attributable risk of 19.2%. In Italy, La Vecchia et al.[58] examined dietary factors and the risk of epithelial ovarian cancer and found that women with the cancer reported significantly increased frequency of consumption of meat (RR = 1.6). In contrast, consumption of fish, green vegetables, carrots, and whole-grain bread or pasta was lower in the cases, and no association with alcohol consumption was found. In an earlier Italian study,[59] positive correlations were also found between gross national internal product and meat consumption, and negative correlations were reported for bread, pasta, or fish consumption.

Some more recent studies of diet and ovarian cancer may shed some different light on the animal fat issue. A case-control study in Greece[60] examined nutrient intakes through the use of a food frequency questionnaire and analyzed them by logistic regression. No substantial, significant associations were found for total energy, total protein, saturated fat, polyunsaturated fat, dietary cholesterol, total carbohydrates, sucrose, vitamins C and A, riboflavin, or calcium. The authors concluded that these results could explain the relatively low incidence of ovarian cancer in Greece and other Mediterranean countries, as well as some of the increasing incidence trends noted in the last few decades.[60] These comments are no doubt in reference to the study by Serra-Majem et al.[61] of mortality trends of breast, colorectal, ovarian, and prostate cancer in Spain, Italy, Greece, Yugoslavia, England, and Wales, which implicated consumption of fat-containing foods in the increase in cancer at these sites in Mediterranean countries, whereas a decrease in ovarian and colorectal cancer was observed

among women in England and Wales. A recent report[62] analyzing 75 epidemiological investigations has concluded that cooked food mutagens may be the
culprit in many of the positive associations seen between meat consumption
and various cancers, although the authors state that the evidence is only strong
for colorectal and not in ovarian cancer. However, it is a mechanism which
may require more careful inquiry on food frequency questionnaires in order to
rule out this dietary component as an etiological factor in cancer of the ovary.

C. Coffee, Lactose, Galactose, and Alcohol

Some unusual dietary variables have been examined for a relationship to
ovarian cancer risk. Two studies[63,64] have reported an association between
coffee drinking and an increased risk of cancer of the ovary, and another one
did not.[52] This subject has been reviewed by Weiss et al.,[65] and the excess risk
appears to be inconsistent among studies. Therefore, the role of coffee as an
etiologic agent in ovarian cancer is not conclusive. A case-control study of
Boston women examined the influence of lactose consumption on the association of oral contraceptive use and ovarian cancer risk.[66] In women who consumed more than 11 g of lactose per day, use of oral contraceptives was
associated with a substantially decreased risk of ovarian cancer (OR = 0.3). The
authors suggest that women who are heavy lactose users may be the most likely
to benefit from the use of oral contraceptives.[66] Interestingly, in another study
of epidemiological aspects of early menopause and ovarian cancer, Cramer[67]
found that galactose consumption through the ingestion of high-lactose dairy
foods may be a dietary risk factor and that galactose metabolism may be a
genetic risk factor for early menopause and ovarian cancer. Cramer[67] suggests
that avoidance of a high-galactose diet may decrease the risk of both early
menopause and ovarian cancer. In contrast, in another case-control study of the
consumption of lactose-containing foods and cancer of the ovary, no differences were found between cases and controls in the frequency of consumption
of dairy foods or in the amount of lactose consumed.[68] A more recent Canadian
case-control study[69] also examined the lactose issue and found that neither
reported history of lactose intolerance nor average daily consumption of lactose
or free galactose was found to be associated with increased risk of ovarian
cancer. The issue of lactose, galactose, and galactose metabolism, therefore,
remains unresolved.

Alcohol and its relation to ovarian cancer risk recently has been examined
by La Vecchia et al.[70] A case-control study of women in the greater Milan,
Italy, area analyzed the consumption of alcohol (90% from wine in this population) and development of ovarian cancer. Relative risks were only modestly
elevated for consumption of over three drinks per day (RR = 1.3), and the
authors concluded that a relatively elevated alcohol intake of 40 g/day or more
resulted in only a modest increase in the incidence of epithelial ovarian cancer.

V. GENERAL CONCLUSIONS, SUMMARY, AND IMPLICATIONS

The genetic basis of familial ovarian cancer with or without breast involvement has been extensively studied. It appears that hereditary ovarian cancer is causally linked to mutations in *BRCA1,* with a cumulative risk by age 70 of 48%. However, few somatic *BRCA1* mutations have been found in sporadic ovarian tumors. The role of *BRCA2* in ovarian cancer is a lesser one in both hereditary and sporadic tumors. As such, however, these genes account for less than 10% of the cases in the population, so other factors obviously must play a role.

Women's general reproductive function such as oral contraceptive use, number of pregnancies, and lactation appear to be somewhat protective. This is speculated to be due to suppression of ovarian function, which may inhibit the cancer development process for epithelial ovarian cancer.

Studies of obesity, height/weight, and body fat distribution have not shown a consistent association with ovarian cancer risk. Specific dietary items which have been positively associated with ovarian cancer are intake of animal fat and meat products. Vegetable consumption appears to be protective. Two studies reported a link between coffee drinking and risk for ovarian cancer, whereas one did not. Only one recent study has reported a modest increase in risk with alcoholic beverage consumption.

The sum of implications from these studies is unfortunately inconclusive. While we can attribute approximately 10% of ovarian cancer cases to mutations in *BRCA1* and *BRCA2*, the vast majority of cases do not have a strong, compelling association with any risk factor, either environmental or dietary. The hormonal influences underlying the development of ovarian cancer need to be better defined, and until we can achieve a better understanding of those mechanisms, the nutritional factors influencing those mechanisms will be poorly understood.

REFERENCES

1. Parker, S.L., Tong, T., Bolden, S., and Wingo, P.A., Cancer statistics 1997, *CA Cancer J. Clin.*, 47, 5, 1997.
2. Cotran, R.S., Kumar, V., and Robbins, S.L., *Robbins Pathologic Basis of Disease*, 5th ed., W.B. Saunders, Philadelphia, 1994, chap. 23.
3. Young, R.H. and Antonioli, D.A., The ovary, in *Diagnostic Surgical Pathology*, Sternberg S., Antonioli, D.A., Carter, D., Mills, S.E., and Oberman, H.A., Eds., Raven Press, New York, 1994, chap. 53.
4. Bell, D.A., Weinstock, M.A., and Scully, R.E., Peritoneal implants of ovarian serous borderline tumors, *Cancer*, 62, 2212, 1988.
5. Watkin, W., Silva, E.G., and Gershenson, D.M., Mucinous carcinoma of the ovary, *Cancer*, 69, 208, 1992.

6. Snyder, R.R., Norris, H.J., and Tavassoli, F., Endometrial proliferative and low malignant potential tumors of the ovary, *Am. J. Surg. Pathol.*, 12, 661, 1988.
7. Bast, R.C., Jacobs, I., and Berchuck, A., Malignant transformation of ovarian epithelium. *J. Natl. Cancer Inst.*, 84, 557, 1992.
8. Shevchuk, M.M., Fenoglio, C.M., and Richart, R.M., Histogenesis of Brenner tumors. I. Histology and ultrastructure. II. Histochemistry and CEA, *Cancer*, 46, 2607, 1980.
9. Linder, D., McCaw, B.K., and Hecht, F., Pathogenetic origin of benign ovarian teratomas, *New Engl. J. Med.*, 292, 63, 1975.
10. Norris, H.J., Zirkin, H.J., and Benson, W.C., Immature (malignant) teratoma of the ovary: a clinical and pathological study of 58 cases, *Cancer*, 37, 2359, 1976.
11. Gordon, T., Lipton, D., and Woodruff, D., Dysgerminoma: a review of 158 cases from the Emil Novak ovarian tumor registry, *Obstet. Gynecol.*, 58, 497, 1981.
12. Teilum, G., *Special Tumors of Ovary and Testis and Relocated Extragonadal Lesions*, W.B. Saunders, Philadelphia, 1976.
13. Young, R.H. and Scully, R., Ovarian sex cord-stromal tumors: recent progress, *Int. J. Gynecol. Pathol.*, 1, 101, 1982.
14. Prat, J. and Scully, R.E., Cellular fibromas and fibrosarcomas of the ovary, *Cancer*, 47, 2663, 1981.
15. Roth, L.M., Anderson, M.C., Govan, A.D.T., Langley, F.A., Gowing, N.F.C., and Woodcock, A.S., Sertoli-Leydig cell tumors: a clinicopathologic study of 34 cases. *Cancer*, 48, 187, 1981.
16. Scully R.E., The ovary, in *Endometrial Pathology*, Wolfe, H., Ed., Springer-Verlag, New York, 1986.
17. Young, R.H. and Scully, R.E., *Metastatic Tumors of the Female Genital Tract*, 4th ed., Springer-Verlag, New York, 1994.
18. DeVita, V.T., Hellman, S., and Rosenberg, S.A., *Cancer: Principles and Practice of Oncology*, 5th ed., Lippincott-Raven Publishers, Philadelphia, 1997, chap. 35.
19. Kerber, R.A. and Slattery, M.L., The impact of family history on ovarian cancer risk. The Utah Population Database, *Arch. Intern. Med.*, 155, 905, 1995.
20. Narod, S.A., Genetics of breast and ovarian cancer, *Br. Med. Bull.*, 50, 656, 1994.
21. Wooster, R., Neuhausen, S., Manigion, J., Quirk, Y., Ford, D., Collins, N., Nguyen, K., Seal, S., Tran, T., Averill, D., Fields, P., Marshall, G., Narod, S., Lenoir, G.M., Lynch, H.T., Feunteun, J., Devilee, P., Cornelisse, C.J., Menko, F.H., Daly, P.A., Ormiston, W., McManus, R., Pye, C., Lewis, C.M., Cannon-Albright, L.A., Peto, J., Ponder, B.A.J., Skolnick, M.H., Easton, D.F., Goldgar, D.E., and Stratton, M.R., Localization of a breast cancer susceptibility gene (*BRCA2*) to chromosome 13q by genetic linkage analysis, *Science*, 265, 2088, 1994.
22. Ford, D. and Easton, D.F., The genetics of breast and ovarian cancer, *Br. J. Cancer*, 72, 805, 1995.
23. Muto, M.G., Cramer, D.W., Tangir, J., Berkowitz, R., and Mok, S., Frequency of the *BRCA1 185delAG* mutation among Jewish women with ovarian cancer and matched population controls, *Cancer Res.*, 56, 1250, 1996.
24. Berman, D.B., Costalas, J., Schultz, D.C., Grano, G., Daly, M., and Godwin, A.K., A common mutation in *BRCA2* that predisposes to a variety of cancers is found in both Jewish Ashkenazi and non-Jewish individuals, *Cancer Res.*, 56, 3409, 1996.

25. Foster, K.A., Harrington, P., Kerr, J., Russell, P., DiCioccio, R.A., Scott, I.V., Jacobs, I., Chenevix-Trench, G., Ponder, B.A.J., and Gayther, S.A., Somatic and germline mutations of the *BRCA2* gene in sporadic ovarian cancer, *Cancer Res.*, 56, 3622, 1996.

26. Watson, P. and Lynch, H.T., Extracolonic cancer in hereditary non-polyposis colorectal cancer, *Cancer*, 71, 677, 1993.

27. Malkin, D., Li, F.P., Strong, L.C., Fraumeni, J.F., Nelson, C.E., Kim, D.H., Kassel, J., Gryka, M.A., Bischoff, F.Z., Tainsky, M.A., and Friend, S.H., Germline *p53* mutations in a familial syndrome of breast cancer, sarcomas and other neoplasms, *Science*, 250, 1233, 1990.

28. Hartmann, L.C., Podratz, K.C., Keeney, G.L., Kamel, N.A., Edmonson, J.H., Grill, J.P., Su, J.Q., Katzmann, J.A., and Roche, P.C., Prognostic significance of *p53* immunostaining in epithelial ovarian cancer, *J. Clin. Oncol.*, 12, 64, 1994.

29. Schwartz, P.E. and Taylor, K.J., Is early detection of ovarian cancer possible? *Ann. Med.*, 25, 519, 1995.

30. Casagrande, J.T., Louie, E.W., Pike, M.C., Roy, S., Ross, R.K., and Henderson, B.E., "Incessant ovulation" and ovarian cancer, *Lancet*, 2, 170, 1979.

31. Cramer, D.W., Hutchison, G.B., Welch, W.R., Scully, R.E., and Knapp, R.C., Factors affecting the association of oral contraceptives and ovarian cancer, *New Engl. J. Med.*, 307, 1047, 1982.

32. Nasca, P.C., Greenwald, P., Chorost, S., Richart, R., and Caputo, T., An epidemiologic case-control study of ovarian cancer and reproductive factors, *Am. J. Epidemiol.*, 119, 705, 1984.

33. Weiss, N.S., Lyon, J.L., Liff, J.M., Vollmer, W.M., and Daling, J.R., Incidence of ovarian cancer in relation to the use of oral contraceptives, *Int. J. Cancer*, 28, 669, 1981.

34. Anon., Epithelial ovarian cancer and combined oral contraceptives. The WHO Collaborative Study of Neoplasia and Steroid Contraceptives, *Int. J. Epidemiol.*, 18, 538, 1989.

35. Gross, T.P., Schlesselman, J.J., Stadel, B.V., Yu, W., and Lee, N.C., The risk of epithelial ovarian cancer in short-term users of oral contraceptives, *Am. J. Epidemiol.*, 136, 46, 1992.

36. Irwin, K.L., Weiss, N.S., and Peterson, H.B., Tubal sterilization, hysterectomy, and the subsequent occurrence of epithelial ovarian cancer, *Am. J. Epidemiol.*, 134, 362, 1991.

37. Mori, M., Harabuchi, I., Miyaki, H., Casagrande, J.T., Henderson, B.E., and Ross, R.K., Reproductive, genetic, and dietary risk factors for ovarian cancer, *Am. J. Epidemiol.*, 128, 771, 1988.

38. Whittemore, A.S., Characteristics relating to ovarian cancer risk: implications for prevention and detection, *Gynecol. Oncol.*, 55, S15, 1994.

39. Rosenblatt, K.A. and Thomas, D.B., Lactation and the risk of epithelial ovarian cancer. The WHO Collaborative Study of Neoplasia and Steroid Contraceptives, *Int. J. Epidemiol.*, 22, 192, 1993.

40. de Mouzon, J., Cohen, J., and Spira, A., Cancer of the ovary and the treatment of infertility: analysis of the article by Whittemore et al., *Contracept. Fertil. Sexualite*, 21, 566, 1993.

41. Gwinn, M.L., Lee, N.C., Rhodes, P.H., Layde, P.M., and Rubin, G.L., Pregnancy, breast-feeding, and oral contraceptives and the risk of epithelial ovarian cancer, *J. Clin. Epidemiol.*, 43, 559, 1990.

42. Anon., Depo-medroxyprogesterone acetate (DMPA) and risk of epithelial ovarian cancer. The WHO Collaborative Study of Neoplasia and Steroid Contraceptives, *Int. J. Cancer*, 49, 191, 1991.

43. John, E.M., Whittemore, A.S., Harris, R., and Itnyre, J., Characteristics relating to ovarian cancer risk: collaborative analysis of seven U.S. case-control studies. Epithelial ovarian cancer in black women, *J. Natl. Cancer Inst.*, 85, 142, 1993.

44. Harlow, B.L. and Hartge, P.A., A review of perineal talc exposure and the risk of ovarian cancer, *Regul. Toxicol. Pharmacol.*, 21, 254, 1995.

45. Annegers, J.F., Strom, H., Decker, D.G., Dockerty, M.B., and O'Fallon, W.M., Ovarian cancer: incidence and case-control study, *Cancer*, 43, 723, 1979.

46. Hildreth, N.G., Kelsey, J.L., LiVolsi, V.A., Fischer, D.B., Holford, T.R., Mostow, E.D., Schwartz, P.E., and White, C., An epidemiologic study of epithelial carcinoma of the ovary, *Am. J. Epidemiol.*, 114, 398, 1981.

47. Lapidus, L., Helgesson, O., Merck, C., and Bjorntorp, P., Adipose tissue distribution and female carcinomas. A 12-year follow-up of participants in the population study of women in Goteborg, Sweden, *Int. J. Obesity*, 12, 361, 1988.

48. Committee on Diet and Health, Food and Nutrition Board, Commission on Life Sciences, National Research Council, *Diet and Health, Implications for Reducing Chronic Disease Risk*, National Academy Press, Washington, D.C., 1989, chap. 22.

49. Barker, D.J., Winter, P.D., Osmond, C., Phillips, D.I., and Sultan, H.Y., Weight gain in infancy and cancer of the ovary, *Lancet*, 345, 1087, 1995.

50. Pukkala, E., Poskioparta, M., Apter, D., and Vihko, V., Life-long physical activity and cancer risk among Finnish female teachers, *Eur. J. Cancer Prev.*, 2, 369, 1993.

51. Cramer, D.W., Welch, W.R., Hutchinson, G.B., Willett, W., and Scully, R.E., Dietary animal fat in relation to ovarian cancer risk, *Obstet. Gynecol.*, 63, 833, 1984.

52. Byers, T., Marshall, J., Graham, S., Mettlin, C., and Swanson, M., A case-control study of dietary and nondietary factors in ovarian cancer, *J. Natl. Cancer Inst.*, 71, 681, 1983.

53. Rose, D.P., Boyar, A.P., and Wynder, E.L., International comparisons of mortality rates for cancer of the breast, ovary, prostate, and colon, and per capita food consumption, *Cancer*, 58, 2363, 1986.

54. Slattery, M.L., Schuman, K.L., West, D.W., French, T.K., and Robison, L.M., Nutrient intake and ovarian cancer, *Am. J. Epidemiol.*, 130, 497, 1989.

55. Shu, X.O., Gao, Y.T., Yuan, J.M., Ziegler, R.G., and Brinton, L.A., Dietary factors and epithelial ovarian cancer, *Br. J. Cancer*, 59, 92, 1989.

56. Kato, I., Tominaga, S., and Kuroishi, T., Relationship between Westernization of dietary habits and mortality from breast and ovarian cancers in Japan, *Jpn. J. Cancer Res.*, 78, 349, 1987.

57. Mori, M. and Miyake, H., Dietary and other risk factors among elderly women, *Jpn. J. Cancer Res.*, 79, 997, 1988.

58. La Vecchia, C., Decarli, A., Negri, E., Parazzini, F., Gentile, A., Cecchetti, G., Fasoli, M., and Franceschi, S., Dietary factors and the risk of epithelial ovarian cancer, *J. Natl. Cancer Inst.*, 79, 663, 1987.

59. Decarli, A. and La Vecchia, C., Environmental factors and cancer mortality in Italy, *Oncology*, 43, 116, 1986.

60. Tzonou, A., Hsieh, C.C., Polychronopoulou, A., Kaprinis, G., Toupadaki, N., Trichopoulou, A., Karakatsani, A., and Trichopoulos, D., Diet and ovarian cancer: a case-control study in Greece, *Int. J. Cancer*, 55, 411, 1993.

61. Serra-Majem, L., La Vecchia, C., Ribas-Barba, L., Prieto-Ramos, F., Lucchini, F., Ramon, J.M., and Salleras, L., Changes in diet and mortality from selected cancers in southern Mediterranean countries, *Eur. J. Clin. Nutr.*, 47, S25, 1993.

62. de Meester, C. and Gerber, G.B., The role of cooked food mutagens as possible etiological agents in human cancer. A critical appraisal of recent epidemiological investigations, *Rev. Epidemiol. Sante Publ.*, 43, 147, 1995.

63. La Vecchia, C., Franceschi, A., Decarli, A., Gentile, P., Liata, M., Regello, M., and Togoni, G., Coffee drinking and risk of epithelial ovarian cancer, *Int. J. Cancer*, 33, 559, 1984.

64. Trichopoulos, D., Papapostolou, M., and Polychronopoulou, A., Coffee and ovarian cancer, *Int. J. Cancer*, 28, 691, 1981.

65. Weiss, N.S., Cook, L.S., Farrow, D.C., and Rosenblatt, K.A., Ovarian cancer, in *Cancer Epidemiology and Prevention*, Schottenfeld, D. and Fraumeni, J.F., Eds., Oxford University Press, New York, 1996, chap. 48.

66. Harlow, B.L., Cramer, D.W., Seller, J., Willett, W.C., Bell, D.A., and Welch, W.R., The influence of lactose consumption on the association of oral contraceptive use and ovarian cancer risk, *Am. J. Epidemiol.*, 134, 445, 1991.

67. Cramer, D.W., Epidemiologic aspects of early menopause and ovarian cancer, *Ann. N.Y. Acad. Sci.*, 592, 363, 1990.

68. Engle, A., Muscat, J.E., and Harris, R.E., Nutritional risk factors and ovarian cancer, *Nutr. Cancer*, 15, 239, 1992.

69. Risch, H.A., Jain, M., Marrett, L.D., and Howe, G.R., Dietary lactose intake, lactose intolerance, and the risk of epithelial ovarian cancer in southern Ontario (Canada), *Cancer Causes Control*, 5, 540, 1994.

70. La Vecchia, C., Negri, E., Franceschi, S., Parazzini, F., Gentile, A., and Fasoli, M., Alcohol and epithelial ovarian cancer, *J. Clin. Epidemiol.*, 45, 1025, 1992.

CHAPTER 5

NUTRITION AND CANCER OF THE ENDOMETRIUM

CONTENTS

I. GENERAL PATHOLOGY AND STATISTICS

Endometrial cancer is the most common invasive cancer of the female genital tract. Endometrial cancer and other nonspecified uterine tumors account for about 6% of all newly diagnosed cancers in women and 2% of all cancer-related deaths.[1] Endometrial hyperplasia is often related to an abnormally high, prolonged level of estrogenic stimulation such as may occur at menopause. It is thought to be a precursor to carcinoma, especially those hyperplasias with cytologic atypia.[2] In fact, about 20% of patients with atypical hyperplasia (cytologic atypia) eventually develop endometrial carcinoma. The peak incidence of endometrial carcinoma is 55–65 years, and it is rare under 40 years of age. It is thought to be associated with prolonged, unopposed estrogen stimulation. Most endometrial carcinoma (about 85%) tends to be adenocarcinoma that presents with postmenopausal bleeding.[3]

Squamous differentiation in the adenocarcinoma is fairly common and is called adenocanthoma. However, if the squamous component is malignant, then the term adenosquamous carcinoma is used.[4,5] The tumor will behave according to stage and grade of the adenocarcinoma component regardless of the absence or presence of squamous differentiation. Two histologic types behave as poorly differentiated despite their degree of differentiation: papillary serous carcinoma and clear cell carcinoma.

Staging of endometrial adenocarcinoma is as follows:[6,7]

Stage I	Carcinoma is confined to the corpus uteri itself
Stage II	Carcinoma has involved the corpus and the cervix
Stage III	Carcinoma has extended outside the uterus but not outside the true pelvis
Stage IV	Carcinoma has extended outside the true pelvis or has obviously involved the mucosa of the bladder or the rectum*

Cases in various stages can also be subgrouped with reference to histologic type of adenocarcinoma as follows:

G1	Well-differentiated adenocarcinoma
G2	Differentiated adenocarcinoma with partly solid areas
G3	Predominantly solid or entirely undifferentiated carcinoma, including all serous and clear cell carcinomas*

Surgery, alone or in combination with irradiation, yields close to 90% 5-year survival in stage I disease. This rate drops to 30–50% in stage II and to less than 20% in any of the other more advanced stages of the disease.

Endometrial stromal tumors are divided into three categories. Benign stromal nodules are well-circumscribed aggregates of endometrial stromal cells in the myometrium. Low-grade stromal sarcoma is also called endolymphatic stromal myosis because it penetrates lymphatic channels. Well-differentiated endometrial stroma lies between myometrial muscle bundles. About 50% recurs after 10–15 years, and metastasis and death occur in 15%. Endometrial stromal sarcoma shows histologically marked atypia with numerous mitoses and is overtly malignant. The 5-year survival rate is about 50%.[5] Malignant

---

* From Cotran, R.S., Kumar, V., and Robbins, S.L., *Robbins Pathologic Basis of Disease*, 5th ed., W.B. Saunders, Philadelphia, 1994, 1062. With permission.

mixed mullerian tumors consist of endometrial adenocarcinomas in which a malignant stromal (mesenchymal) component develops. The tumors are highly malignant and have a 5-year survival rate of about 25%.[8-10]

II. POPULATION GENETICS AND MARKERS FOR RISK

A. Replication Error Phenotype

Endometrial carcinoma is primarily a disease of postmenopausal women in which perimenopausal anovulation results in a deficiency of progesterone and thus an unopposed estrogen state.[11] The influence of unopposed estrogen results in cell proliferation leading to endometrial hyperplasia. As genetic damage accumulates, this hyperplasia degenerates to an atypical hyperplasia, which can be regarded as a precursor of endometrial carcinoma. Epidemiologic studies have shown that endometrial cancer is more common in women with either prior malignancies of the breast, colon, and ovary or in those with family histories of colon cancer. One such syndrome is Lynch syndrome II or hereditary nonpolyposis colon cancer (HNPCC).[12] Henry Lynch has stated that "the most significant genetic association of endometrial cancer occurs with HNPCC of the Lynch II variant." This variant shows all the features of the Lynch I syndrome HNPCC, but also the presence of other cancers, particularly predisposition to endometrial cancer. A recent study has implicated microsatellite heterogeneities in endometrial cancer from patients having a history of HNPCC.[13] The "replication error" (RER+) phenotype is characterized by instability of dinucleotide repeat sequences throughout the genome, known as microsatellite instability.[13] Risinger et al.[13] also observed microsatellite instability in 17% of sporadic endometrial carcinoma and in 75% of those tumors associated with HNPCC, indicating that the HNPCC gene is involved in both heritable and somatic forms of endometrial cancer. Carduff et al.[14] have further examined the clinical and pathological significance of microsatellite instability in sporadic endometrial cancer. They found microsatellite instability in 9% of the endometrial cancers studied, and this was significantly associated with a high histological grade and adverse outcome. The authors concluded that the RER+ phenotype is only present in a minority of sporadic endometrial cancers, as opposed to those associated with HNPCC. These conclusions confirmed those reported by Katabuchi et al.,[15] who performed mutational analyses of four mismatch repair genes in sporadic endometrial cancer having an RER+ phenotype and concluded that mutations in known DNA mismatch repair genes are not responsible for most of the microsatellite instability seen in those sporadic endometrial tumors which display the RER+ phenotype. In contrast, Duggan et al.[16] have reported the presence of the RER+ phenotype in 20% of sporadic endometrial cancers. The authors concluded that the RER+ phenotype is frequently present in sporadic endometrial cancer and that it is expressed before and during clonal expansion of the transformed cells and is limited to neoplastic tissue only.

B. Oncogene Mutations

Oncogenes of the *ras* family have been shown to be either mutated or overexpressed in endometrial carcinoma.[17–20] Ignar-Trowbridge et al.[18] found these Ki-*ras* mutations in codon 12 in 10% of endometrial cancers. Mizuuchi et al.[19] have suggested that the Ki-*ras* protooncogene activation plays an important role in the determination of the aggressiveness of endometrial cancer. Sato et al.[20] have concluded that there is no correlation between *ras* mutations and stage and grade of histological differentiation in endometrial cancer. Likewise, Carduff et al.[21] also found no correlation between the prevalence of Ki-*ras* mutations with stage, grade, or clinical outcome of endometrial cancer. However, in contrast, Sasaki et al.[22] reported that Ki-*ras* mutation was an early event in some endometrial cancers and that the presence of this mutation was inversely associated with death from the disease. Therefore, it can be concluded that activated *ras* genes may be responsible for the development of a small percentage of endometrial tumors.

Other oncogenes which may play a role in endometrial cancer are c-*myc* and the epidermal growth factor receptor, as well as the Her-2/neu oncogene.[23] More recently, the *p53* gene product has been examined in endometrial carcinomas and found to be overexpressed in 21% of tumors.[24] In addition to *p53* mutations, genes residing on chromosomes 1, 3, 6, 11, 13, 15, 17, 18, 20, 21, and X have demonstrated the presence of nonrandom allelic deletions and abnormalities.[25] Kohler et al.[26] reported that the mutation of *p53* was not found in endometrial hyperplasias and concluded that *p53* mutations may be a relatively late event in endometrial cancer. Kihana et al.[27] examined the presence of *p53* mutations in endometrial cancer in reference to clinical outcome. The authors concluded from their study of loss of heterozygosity and mutations in 92 patients that the loss of heterozygosity patients had a poorer postoperative survival and that patients with both loss of heterozygosity and mutations had the worst prognosis. They suggest that the *p53* gene may play an important role in the development of endometrial cancer. It is certain that more research is needed into the genes that might play a role in endometrial cancer.

III. GENERAL EPIDEMIOLOGY OF ENDOMETRIAL CANCER

A. Exogenous Unopposed Estrogens

As stated above, endometrial cancer has been correlated with cancers of the breast, ovary, colon, and rectum.[28] It has also been found to be significantly associated with cutaneous malignant melanomas as a second primary cancer,[29] with a standardized incidence ratio of 1.41. It tends to be more common in the United States than in other parts of the world and is more frequent in Caucasian women of higher socioeconomic status. The major established etiologic cause for this cancer appears to be the use of exogenous estrogens at the high doses commonly prescribed years ago.[30] In contrast, postmenopausal hormone replacement therapy containing progestins has been associated with a lower risk of endometrial cancer than therapy with estrogens alone.[31,32] Decreased risks have also been observed in association with the use of combination-type oral contraceptives,[33] suggesting that overall the risk is specifically related to estrogen exposure that is unopposed by progestins.[34] Recent findings[35] suggest that combined oral contraceptives with varying doses of estrogen and progestin may have different effects on the risk for endometrial cancer depending on the doses of each used. Hulka[36] has reviewed the links between hormone replacement therapy and neoplasia. She has concluded from her review that the doses commonly used for estrogen replacement therapy are sufficient to cause proliferation, hyperplasia, and carcinoma of the endometrium, and the result is that after 10–15 years of use, endometrial cancer risk is increased tenfold. However, she notes that these cancers are generally of low grade and stage with an excellent prognosis. But the addition of progestin to the regimen at least 10 days per month reduces or eliminates the increased risk associated with estrogen therapy.[36] However, a number of other potential risk factors have surfaced in recent years that may put a new angle on the estrogen hypothesis.

B. Intrauterine Devices, Breast-Feeding, and Pregnancy

Parazzini et al.[37] have studied the relationship between intrauterine device (IUD) use and the risk of endometrial cancer in a case-control study in Italian women. Their results suggest a protective effect of IUD use on endometrial cancer, but also suggest caution in interpretation due to possible indication bias.

Since it is widely understood that the risk of endometrial cancer is related to estrogen levels, there is a suggestion that during breast-feeding, because the reduction of estrogen is greater than that of progesterone, lactation might reduce the risk of endometrial cancer. Rosenblatt and Thomas[38] examined this hypothesis in data from six countries in a hospital-based case-control study. Through questionnaires, they assessed the impact of breast-feeding duration and the age at which the lactation was started and stopped. They reported a significant decreasing trend in risk with increasing duration of lactation and with months of breast-feeding per pregnancy.[38] The apparent protective effect declined with time since cessation of breast-feeding, so that there was no evidence of a protective effect past age 55, the age at which this disease is most prevalent. Therefore, the impact of this practice on overall risk of endometrial cancer would appear to be minimal.

In the Iowa Women's Health Study, McPherson et al.[39] found that gravidity was a risk factor for endometrial cancer. In 5 years of follow-up, the authors reported that the mean gravidity of cases was lower than that of controls (2.3 vs. 3.5, P <0.001). They concluded that these and other findings from this study support the "unopposed" estrogen hypothesis for the etiology of endometrial cancer.

C. Ovarian Dysfunction

Ovarian dysfunction has been reported as a risk factor for endometrial cancer in younger women. A Swedish study[40] reported that among other known risk factors such as hirsutism, increased body mass index, and hypertension, there was also an association with untreated ovarian dysfunction, such as is present in polycystic ovarian disease. This was only seen in younger women with endometrial cancer and is thought to be associated with the unopposed estrogen action on the endometrium that is seen in this disorder.

An interesting variation on this hypothesis is the observation first reported in 1992 by Persson et al.[41] that there was a reduced risk of hip fracture in women with endometrial cancer. This was thought to be consistent with the hypothesis that the persistent influence of endogenous estrogens was responsible for both the endometrial cancer and the reduction in risk of hip fractures. Extending this work, Persson et al.[42] later reported that there was a reduced risk of breast and endometrial cancer among women with hip fractures. The authors suggest that these results are consistent with the hypothesis that long-term estrogen deficiency is associated with a decreased risk of developing breast or endometrial cancer.

D. Cholesterol, Diabetes, and Hypertension

Blood lipids have been studied in a multicenter case-control study that included 256 cases of endometrial cancer and 185 controls, all of whom were less than 75 years old.[43] Blood lipids including serum cholesterol, LDL and HDL cholesterol, and triglycerides were generally lower in cases compared with controls. After adjusting for age, education, smoking status, obesity, and body fat distribution, the relative risks for endometrial cancer increased (P for trend <0.01) across decreasing quartiles of serum cholesterol (relative risks = 1.0, 2.5, 2.4, and 4.2), and the authors could not rule out hypocholesterolemia as a risk factor for endometrial cancer.[43]

The risk of endometrial cancer in diabetics and hypertensives has been studied in 1715 Finnish women diagnosed during 1970–74 with cancer of the endometrium.[44] Data from the insurance register linked them to diagnoses for diabetes and/or hypertension. Diabetes was found to be a strong, and hypertension a relatively weak, risk factor for endometrial cancer.[44] The relative risk for diabetes was 4.1 and for hypertension was 1.6, and these are now considered to be identifiable risk factors for endometrial cancer in Finland. No obvious biological explanation is available at this time. Another recent case-control study of diabetes mellitus and cancer risk in Italy[45] reported that significantly elevated relative risks were found for cancer of the endometrium (3.4) and liver (2.8). After adjustments for obesity, education, age, and sex, the relative risk was 3.0 for liver cancer and 2.8 for cancer of the endometrium. The elevated risks remained for up to 10 years after a diagnosis of diabetes mellitus.

E. Conjugated Estrogens and Tamoxifen

The relationship between the use of unopposed estrogens and endometrial cancer has been studied in a southern California population of 318 patients from the Kaiser Foundation Health Plan.[46] They were compared with 599 controls matched for age and duration of membership in the prepaid health plan. A history of the use of conjugated estrogens and users vs. nonusers was contrasted. The authors found that estrogen-induced risk of endometrial cancer decreases rapidly as the estrogen-free time interval increases.[46] The risk ratio decreased from 5.0 for those who had discontinued use less than 24 months prior to the diagnosis down to 1.8 for a time interval since use between 24 and 48 months, and for greater than 48 months the ratio was near 1.[46] These results indicate that discontinuation of the use of unopposed estrogens significantly decreases risk for endometrial cancer in a time-dependent manner.

Since the drug tamoxifen is being increasingly used worldwide for the treatment of breast cancer, Rutqvist et al.[47] examined the carcinogenic risks among 2729 Stockholm women on long-term use of tamoxifen. After a median follow-up of 9 years, the tamoxifen-treated patients demonstrated a sixfold increase in endometrial cancer ($P < 0.001$) and a threefold increase in gastrointestinal cancers. The relative risk associated with tamoxifen use for endometrial cancer was 4.1, 1.9 for colorectal cancer, and 3.2 for stomach cancer.[47] These data indicate that there is a need for extensive surveillance of women who are taking tamoxifen in the Breast Cancer Prevention Trial for the development of these other malignancies. A recent study of women at the Roswell Park Cancer Institute[48] with both breast and endometrial cancer who were using tamoxifen has determined that the maximum estimate of endometrial cancer risk is 2 of 402 cases or 0.05%. Therefore, these authors conclude that the risk of endometrial cancer with tamoxifen use is low and that the value of routine invasive screening for endometrial cancer for women receiving tamoxifen should be determined by an in-depth prospective study.

Although endometrial cancer has been regarded as a disease associated with excessive exposure to exogenous estrogens, Potischman et al.[49] have recently examined in a case-control study the risk associated with the circulating levels of steroid hormones and sex hormone binding globulin (SHBG). This study involved both premenopausal and postmenopausal women and excluded women who reported use of exogenous estrogens within 6 months of the interview.

Blood samples were collected and analyzed for circulating steroid hormones and SHBG. Results demonstrated that high levels of androstenedione were associated with 3.6-fold and 2.8-fold increased risks among premenopausal and postmenopausal women, respectively, and a reduced risk among postmenopausal women was related to high SHBG levels. A higher risk was associated with high estrone levels (odds ratio = 3.8), as was albumin-bound estrogen (odds ratio = 2.2), but only in postmenopausal women. In contrast, premenopausal women showed no increased risk with high circulating levels of total, free, and albumin-bound estrogen. The authors conclude that there should be further research on alternate hormonal mechanisms for the risk associated with obesity and body fat distribution and that the role of androstenedione should be more extensively evaluated.

The role of cigarette smoking in endometrial cancer has been studied extensively, and the studies have generally found that smokers are at a reduced risk for this malignancy, thought to be due to the observation that smokers have reduced premenopausal urinary excretion of endogenous estrogens and menopause at a younger age.[50] A recent case-control study of this phenomenon showed that cigarette smokers were at reduced risk of endometrial cancer (relative risk = 0.6) and that current smokers demonstrated the greatest reduction in risk (relative risk = 0.4), with both effects apparently confined to postmenopausal women.[50]

IV. OBESITY, BODY WEIGHT, AND BODY FAT DISTRIBUTION

A. Body Mass Correlations

Many epidemiological studies have examined the relationship between the risk of endometrial cancer and body weight, obesity, and fat distribution patterns, and a number have shown that the risk of endometrial cancer increases considerably with increasing weight (Table 5.1).[51,52] Generally, obesity has been cited as a risk factor in a number of studies,[53–57] and a hormonally based mechanism has been postulated for this association. Additionally, in a case-control study in China,[58] obesity also proved to be a strong risk factor for endometrial cancer, even in a country where supplemental estrogen use is uncommon. However, another study[59] has shown no association between obesity and endometrial cancer. A case-control study of endometrial adenocarcinoma in Athens, Greece, investigated the epidemiology of this cancer in a low-risk setting,[59] and no relationship was found between body weight and endometrial cancer. There also appears to be an association between endometrial cancer risk and body fat distribution, with certain studies demonstrating that women with more upper body fat have an increased risk of endometrial cancer.[60] A longitudinal population study of 1462 women in Sweden[61] exam-

Table 5.1   Studies of Body Mass, Body Fat, and Risk of Endometrial Cancer

Factor	Type of Study	Association with Risk	Reference
Body weight	Case-control	Increased risk	Parazzini et al.[51]
	Cohort, prospective	Increased risk	Folsom et al.[52]
Obesity	Varied	Increased risk	Elwood et al.[53]
			Henderson et al.[54]
			La Vecchia et al.[55]
			Lew and Garfinkel[56]
			Wynder et al.[57]
	Case-control	Strong risk, odds ratio = 2.5	Shu et al.[58]
	Case-control	No association	Koumantaki et al.[59]
Body weight	Case-control	No association	Koumantaki et al.[59]
Upper body fat	Case-control	Increased risk	Schapira[60]
Abdominal fat	Cohort, prospective	Increased risk	Lapidus et al.[61]
Body mass index	Case-control	Increased risk in 30s and 50s	Levi et al.[62]
	Case-control	Increased risk; obesity age 16	Olson et al.[63]
	Case-control	Increased risk	Swanson et al.[64]

ined adipose tissue distribution and the occurrences of endometrial cancer and reported that abdominally localized adipose tissue was associated with irregular ovulation and menstruation, as well as an increased risk of endometrial cancer.

Body mass index (BMI) at different ages and subsequent risk of endometrial cancer was studied in a multicenter case-control study of women in Switzerland and northern Italy.[62] The results indicated that in women who were normal weight at diagnosis, there was no significant effect of past overweight. However, in those who were overweight at the time of diagnosis of their cancer, there were significant relationships with BMI in the third and fifth decades of life. The authors suggest that to lower endometrial cancer risk, women must avoid obesity in later middle and older age.[62] Similar findings of an association between endometrial cancer and excess weight at 16 years of age and larger gains over time up to the time of diagnosis were reported by Olson et al.[63] in women in western New York. Thus, it appears that weight control after puberty is important in reducing the risk of endometrial cancer postmenopausally.

A recent report examined in a case-control study of 403 endometrial cancer cases and 297 controls the relationship of past and contemporary body size, including body fat distribution, to risk for endometrial cancer.[64] Height was not found to be a risk factor, but sitting height was inversely associated with risk. Women with measured weight above 78 kg had a 2.3-fold increase in risk compared with those who weighed less than 58 kg.[64] Contemporary weight gain as weight gained during adulthood was also seen as a separate risk factor. Upper body obesity was a risk factor independent of body weight, and the relative risks across increasing quartiles of upper body obesity were 1.0, ,1.5, 1.8, and 2.6. These results appear to support the contention that both obesity and adipose tissue distribution increase the risk for endometrial cancer.

B. Physical Activity

Also relevant to the role of obesity in endometrial cancer is the association of this cancer with physical activity. Levi et al.[65] examined the relationship between various indicators of physical activity and endometrial cancer risk in a case-control study in Switzerland and Italy. Their data showed that a moderate or high level of physical activity was an indicator of reduced endometrial cancer risk, although further evaluation of these findings is warranted. Another study of physical activity and risk for endometrial cancer[66] reported that women who led basically sedentary lifestyles were at somewhat increased risk; however, the lack of elevation in risk among women who were physically inactive outside of occupational activity tends to weaken the association.

V. DIETARY FAT, FRUITS, AND VEGETABLES

In assessing the effects of particular dietary factors and endometrial cancer (Table 5.2), one of the first studies was performed in Italy[55] in which a case-control study collected data on the frequency of consumption of selected dietary items. The cases with endometrial cancer reported a greater fat intake and a less frequent intake of fruits, vegetables, and grains. A subsequent study by the same investigators[67] examined Italian regional diets and their correlation to breast, ovarian, and endometrial cancer rates. Diets high in fat, protein, and calories increased the incidence rates of all three cancers, and diets high in

Table 5.2   Studies of Dietary Fat, Fruits and Vegetables, and Risk of Endometrial Cancer

Nutrient/Factor	Type of Study	Association with Risk	Reference
Fat	Case-control	Increased risk	La Vecchia et al.[55]
Fat, oleic acid	Case-control	Increased risk	Potischman et al.[71]
Fat, protein, calories	Case-control	Increased risk	La Vecchia[67]
Cholesterol	Case-control	Increased risk	Barbone et al.[70]
Calories	Case-control	Increased, odds ratio = 2.1	Shu et al.[68]
Energy intake, meats	Case-control	Increased risk	Levi et al.[69]
Energy, animal foods	Cohort, prospective	No association	Zheng et al.[73]
Fruits and vegetables	Case-control	Decreased risk	La Vecchia et al.[55]
	Case-control	Decreased risk	La Vecchia[67]
	Case-control	No association	Potischman et al.[71]
Fruits and allium sp.	Case-control	Decreased risk	Shu et al.[68]
Carotene, nitrate	Case-control	Decreased risk	Barbone et al.[70]
Fruits, vegetables, grains	Case-control	Decreased risk	Levi et al.[69]
Breads and cereals	Case-control	Decreased risk	Potischman et al.[71]
Processed meat, fish	Cohort, prospective	Increased risk	Zheng et al.[73]
Cooked food mutagens	Review of studies	No conclusions	de Meester and Gerber[72]

green vegetable and fresh fruit consumption had a protective effect. The relation between diet and endometrial cancer has also been examined in China.[68] Women in the highest quartile of total caloric intake had a 2.1-fold increased risk of endometrial cancer, and that risk varied according to the source of calories, with the highest risk attributable to caloric intake, although fruit and allium vegetables were associated with some reduction in risk.[68] A more recent study of women in Switzerland and northern Italy[69] found significant direct associations with the total energy intake and the frequency of consumption of most types of meats, eggs, beans or peas, added fats, and sugar. Significant protection or decreased risk was seen in the highest vs. the lowest consumption tertile for most vegetables, fresh fruits, and whole grains.[69]

In a case-control study of diet and endometrial cancer conducted in Birmingham, Alabama,[70] a high intake of certain micronutrients was found to be associated with a decreased risk of endometrial cancer for those in the upper tertile of carotene and nitrate intake. There was also an inverse association between endometrial cancer and protein consumption, as well as a direct association with cholesterol intake. More frequent consumption of several vegetables and certain dairy products was associated with a statistically significant decreased risk of endometrial cancer.[70] These data were further substantiated by Potischman et al.[71] in a case-control study of women in the United States. They reported increased risk for endometrial cancer associated with higher intakes of fat, with slightly stronger associations with saturated fat and oleic acid than for linoleic acid.[71] Intake of complex carbohydrates, especially breads and cereals, was associated with reduced risks, and these were independent of each other. No consistent relationships were noted for the intakes of cholesterol, fiber, vitamins A and C, specific carotenoids, or foods rich in folate. These data implicate dietary fat/animal fat and low intake of complex carbohydrates in the etiology of endometrial cancer.[71] The authors concluded that these findings are consistent with the hormonal hypothesis for endometrial cancer, but were independent of obesity as a risk factor. Dietary associations have been further specified in a French study which investigated the role of cooked food mutagens as possible etiological agents in human cancer,[72] and the authors concluded that from the studies of all cancers, the pyrolysis products generated from the heat treatment of protein-rich food could be responsible for colorectal cancer. Too few studies were available for any conclusions to be drawn about endometrial cancer and the preference for well-browned meat. Zheng et al.[73] reported no statistical association between dietary intake of energy and most animal foods with endometrial cancer in the prospective Iowa Women's Health Study of over 23,000 postmenopausal women answering a mailed questionnaire. However, they did discern a 50% excess risk associated with the highest tertile of consumption of processed meat and fish, compared with the lowest tertile. These results taken together suggest that animal fat and protein may play a role in the etiology of endometrial cancer, but that the data are not extensive enough to support a role for cooking preference in this etiology.

VI. ALCOHOL CONSUMPTION

Not as much has been published on the relationship between endometrial cancer risk and alcoholic beverage consumption. Two studies have noted an inverse association between alcohol and risk of endometrial cancer,[74,75] but these studies have been criticized for not adequately dealing with confounding and inappropriate choice of controls. A later study[76] addressed the shortcomings of the previous reports and found in their case-control study of women younger than 55 years of age that the risk of endometrial cancer decreased with increasing levels of alcohol intake. Women who consumed an average of ten drinks per week had 50% of the risk of abstainers.[76] However, in contrast, an Italian study[55] reported that women who consumed alcoholic beverages had increased risk for endometrial cancer. The most recent investigation into this phenomenon was a multicenter case-control study in U.S. women[77] which examined the adulthood average weekly intake of beer, wine, and liquor in terms of endometrial cancer risk. A weak protective effect (relative risk = 0.82) was found in women who drank compared with those who never imbibed. The effect was predominantly seen in younger women (<55) where the relative risks were 0.78, 0.64, and 0.41 for increasing levels of alcohol consumption compared with nondrinkers.[77] These results suggest that there may be an inverse association between alcohol consumption and risk for endometrial cancer, but the authors are cautious about causality, although alcohol intake is reported to increase SHBG[78] to decrease serum estrogen.[79]

Although the issue of alcohol intake and endometrial cancer has been studied predominantly in case-control studies, the association between alcohol and endometrial cancer has also been studied prospectively in the Iowa Women's Health Study in the United States.[80] The authors found no association between alcohol consumption and endometrial cancer risk and no interaction with other risk factors such as BMI or estrogen replacement therapy. These authors further conclude that their data do not support an etiologic role for alcohol consumption and endometrial cancer among postmenopausal women.

VII. GENERAL CONCLUSIONS, SUMMARY, AND IMPLICATIONS

In summarizing the genetic information related to endometrial cancer, it appears that there is some genetic component associated with this cancer, but no target gene for predisposition has been identified. The predominant risk factor for cancer of the uterine corpus appears to be "unopposed" estrogenic stimulation of endometrial tissue, due either to endogenous factors or an exogenous source of the hormones. Whether these endogenous factors are genetically controlled or more environmentally influenced cannot be determined at this time.

The inverse connection between cigarette smoking and endometrial cancer is intriguing, but is not to be considered seriously as an intervention to reduce risk, since the other health risks associated with cigarette smoking far outweigh any potential benefits to be gained. Likewise, there may also be an inverse association between alcoholic beverage consumption and endometrial cancer risk, although these data must be interpreted cautiously as to cause and effect. The hormonal effects of alcohol ingestion on SHBG and serum estrogen levels appear to be beneficial; however, more research is needed into this phenomenon.

Body weight, obesity, BMI, and body fat distribution all appear to be risk factors for endometrial cancer, and the consensus of the literature cited supports this contention. This subject has been reviewed recently by Hill and Austin.[81] However, the thought is still that the effects of these variables are ultimately operating through estrogen metabolism and overexposure, still consistent with an "unopposed" estrogen hypothesis. More research is needed on the interactions between hormonal status, these nutritionally related factors, and endometrial cancer risk within the same study population.

Dietary variables such as fat, fruits, and vegetables all seem to point to a trend for increased risk associated with fat intake, meat protein, and total calories in general. There appears to be a role for increased consumption of fruits and vegetables in decreasing risk. However, the data do not point to any specific vitamin as being protective. Again, these conclusions are also consistent with a hormonal hypothesis for endometrial cancer in that dietary fat may contribute to increased estrogen exposure, either through a direct effect on estrogen metabolism or due to its contribution to obesity.

The implications for reduction of risk for endometrial cancer appear to be inextricably intertwined with hormone status, both endogenous and exogenous. Therefore, it would appear that any future studies of nutritional factors and this cancer should focus on the effects of certain nutrients on hormone status and that case-control studies should attempt to correlate nutrient intake with hormonal status in order to determine a mechanistic link.

REFERENCES

1. Parker, S.L., Tong, T., Bolden, S., and Wingo, P.A., Cancer statistics 1997, *CA Cancer J. Clin.*, 47, 5, 1997.
2. Brinton, L.A., Berman, M.L., Mortel, R., Twiggs, L.B., Barrett, R.J., Wilbanks, G.D., Lannom, L., and Hoover, R.N., Reproductive, menstrual, and medical risk factors for endometrial cancer: results from a case-control study, *Am. J. Obstet. Gynecol.*, 167, 1317, 1992.
3. Connelly, P.J., Alberhasky, R.C., and Christopherson, W.M., Carcinoma of the endometrium. III. Analysis of 865 cases of adenocarcinoma and adenocanthoma. *Obstet. Gynecol.*, 59, 569, 1982.

4. Hendrickson, M.R., Schwartz, P.F., and Vidone, R.A., Adenocarcinoma of the endometrium: analysis of 256 cases with disease limited to uterine corpus. Analysis of prognostic variables, *Gynecol. Oncol.*, 12, 373, 1982.

5. Silverberg, S.G. and Kurman, R.J., *Atlas of Tumor Pathology. Tumors of the Uterine Corpus and Gestational Trophoblastic Disease*, Armed Forces Institute of Pathology, Washington, D.C., 1991, 219.

6. Cowles, T.A., Magrina, J.F., Masterson, B.J., and Capen, C.V., Comparison of clinical and surgical staging in patients with endometrial carcinoma, *Obstet. Gynecol.*, 66, 413, 1985.

7. Cotran, R.S., Kumar, V., and Robbins, S.L., *Robbins Pathologic Basis of Disease*, 5th ed., W.B. Saunders, Philadelphia, 1994, chap. 23.

8. Christpherson, W.M. and Richardson, M., Uterine mesenchymal tumors, *Pathol. Ann.*, 16, 215, 1981.

9. Geisinger, K.R., Dabbs, D.J., and Marshall, R.B., Malignant mixed mullerian tumors: an ultrastructural and immunohistochemical analysis with histogenetic considerations, *Cancer*, 54, 1281, 1987.

10. Silverberg, S.G., Major, F.J., Blessing, J.A., Fetter, B., Askin, F.B., Liao, S.-Y., and Miller, A., Carcinosarcoma (malignant mixed mesodermal tumor of the uterus), *Int. J. Gynecol. Pathol.*, 9, 1, 1990.

11. Taylor, R.R., Teneriello, M.G., Nash, J.D., Park, R.C., and Birrer, M.J., The molecular genetics of gynecologic malignancies, *Oncology*, 8, 63, 1994.

12. Lynch, H.T., Lynch, J.F., Conway, T.A., and Bewtra, C., Genetics and gynecologic cancer, in *Principles and Practice of Gynecologic Oncology*, Hoskins, W.J., Perez, C.A., and Young, R.C., Eds., J.B. Lippincott, Philadelphia, 1992, 27.

13. Risinger, J.L., Berchuck, A., Kohler, M.F., Watson, P., Lynch, H.T., and Boyd, J., Genetic instability of microsatellites in endometrial carcinoma, *Cancer Res.*, 53, 5100, 1993.

14. Carduff, R.F., Johnston, C.M., Svoboda-Newman, S.M., Poy, E.L., Merajver, S.D., and Frank, T.S., Clinical and pathological significance of microsatellite instability in sporadic endometrial carcinoma, *Am. J. Pathol.*, 148, 1671, 1996.

15. Katabuchi, H., van Rees, B., Lambers, A.R., Ronnett, B.M., Blazes, M.S., Leach, F.S., Cho, K.R., and Hedrick, L., Mutations in the DNA mismatch repair genes are not responsible for microsatellite instability in most endometrial carcinomas, *Cancer Res.*, 55, 5556, 1995.

16. Duggan, B.D., Felix, J.C., Muderspach, L.I., Tourgemain, D., Zhang, J., and Shibata, D., Microsatellite instability in sporadic endometrial carcinoma, *J. Natl. Cancer Inst.*, 86, 1216, 1994.

17. Long, C.A., O'Brien, T.J., Sanders, M.M., Bard, D.S., and Quirk, J.G., *ras* oncogene is expressed in adenocarcinoma of the endometrium, *Am. J. Obstet. Gynecol.*, 159, 1512, 1988.

18. Ignar-Trowbridge, D., Risinger, J.I., Dent, G.A., Kohler, M., Berchuck, A., McLachlan, J.A., and Boyd, J., Mutations of the Ki-*ras* oncogene in endometrial carcinoma, *Am. J. Obstet. Gynecol.*, 167, 227, 1992.

19. Mizuuchi, H., Nasim, S., Kudo, R., Silverberg, S.G., Greenhouse, S., and Garrett, C.T., Clinical implications of K-*ras* mutations in malignant epithelial tumors of the endometrium, *Cancer Res.*, 52, 2777, 1992.

20. Sato, S., Ito, K., Ozawa, N., Yajima, A., and Sasano, H., Analysis of point mutations at codon 12 of K-*ras* in human endometrial carcinoma and cervical

adenocarcinoma by dot blot hybridization and polymerase chain reaction, *Tohoku J. Exp. Med.*, 165, 131, 1991.

21. Carduff, R.F., Johnston, C.M., and Frank, T.S., Mutations of the Ki-*ras* oncogene in carcinoma of the endometrium, *Am. J. Pathol.*, 146, 182, 1995.

22. Sasaki, H., Nishii, H., Takahashi, H., Tada, A., Furusato, M., Terashima, Y., Siegal, G.P., Parker, S.L., Kohler, M.F., Berchuck, A., and Boyd, J., Mutation of the Ki-*ras* protooncogene in human endometrial hyperplasia and carcinoma, *Cancer Res.*, 53, 1906, 1993.

23. Sato, S., Ito, K., Ozawa, N., Yajima, A., and Sasano, H., Expression of c-*myc*, epidermal growth factor receptor and c-*erb*B-2 in human endometrial carcinoma and cervical adenocarcinoma, *Tohoku J. Exp. Med.*, 165, 137, 1991.

24. Kohler, M.F., Berchuck, A., Davidoff, A.M., Humphrey, P.A., Dodge, R.K., Iglehart, J.D., Soper, J.T., Clarke-Rearson, D.L., Bast, R.C., Jr., and Marks, J.R., Overexpression and mutation of *p53* in endometrial carcinoma, *Cancer Res.*, 52, 1622, 1992.

25. Okamoto, A., Sameshima, Y., Yamada, Y., Teshima, S., Terashima, Y., Terada, M., and Yokota, J., Allelic loss on chromosome 17p and *p53* mutations in human endometrial carcinoma of the uterus, *Cancer Res.*, 51, 5632, 1991.

26. Kohler, M.F., Nishii, H., Humphrey, P.A., Marks, J., Bast, R.C., Clarke-Pearson, D.L., Boyd, J., and Berchuck, A., Mutation of the *p53* tumor-suppressor gene is not a feature of endometrial hyperplasia, *Am. J. Obstet. Gynecol.*, 169, 690, 1993.

27. Kihana, T., Hamada, K., Inoue, Y., Yano, N., Iketani, H., Murao, S., Ukita, M., and Matsuura, S., Mutation and allelic loss of the *p53* gene in endometrial carcinoma: incidence and outcome in 92 surgical patients, *Cancer*, 76, 72, 1995.

28. Miller, A.B., An overview of hormone-associated cancers, *Cancer Res.*, 38, 3985, 1978.

29. Wassberg, C., Thorn, M., Yuen, J., Ringborg, U., and Hakulinen, T., Second primary cancers in patients with cutaneous malignant melanoma: a population-based study in Sweden, *Br. J. Cancer*, 73, 255, 1996.

30. Committee on Diet and Health, Food and Nutrition Board, Commission on Life Sciences, National Research Council, *Diet and Health, Implications for Reducing Chronic Disease Risk*, National Academy Press, Washington, D.C., 1989, chap. 22.

31. Voight, L.F., Weiss, N.S., Chu, J., Daling, J.R., McKnight, B., and van Belle, G., Progestogen supplementation of exogenous oestrogens and risk of endometrial cancer, *Lancet*, 338, 274, 1991.

32. Brinton, L.A. and Hoover, R.N., Estrogen replacement therapy and endometrial cancer risk: unresolved issues. The Endometrial Cancer Collaborative Group, *Obstet. Gynecol.*, 81, 265, 1993.

33. Voight, L.F., Deng, Q., and Weiss, N.S., Recency, duration, and progestin content of oral contraceptives in relation to the incidence of endometrial cancer (Washington, USA), *Cancer Causes Control*, 5, 227, 1994.

34. Key, T.J. and Pike, M.C., The dose–effect relationship between "unopposed" oestrogens and endometrial mitotic rate: its central role in predicting endometrial cancer risk, *Br. J. Cancer*, 57, 205, 1988.

35. Rosenblatt, K.A. and Thomas, D.B., Hormonal content of combined oral contraceptives in relation to the reduced risk of endometrial carcinoma. The WHO

Collaborative Study of Neoplasia and Steroid Contraceptives, *Int. J. Cancer*, 49, 870, 1991.

36. Hulka, B.S., Links between hormone replacement therapy and neoplasia, *Fertil. Steril.*, 62, 1685, 1994.

37. Parazzini, F., La Vecchia, C., and Moroni, S., Intrauterine device use and risk of endometrial cancer, *Br. J. Cancer*, 70, 672, 1994.

38. Rosenblatt, K.A. and Thomas, D.B., Prolonged lactation and endometrial cancer. WHO Collaborative Study of Neoplasia and Steroid Contraceptives, *Int. J. Epidemiol.*, 24, 499, 1995.

39. McPherson, C.P., Sellers, T.A., Potter, J.D., Bostick, R.M., and Folsom, A.R., Reproductive factors and risk of endometrial cancer: the Iowa Women's Health Study, *Am. J. Epidemiol.*, 143, 1195, 1996.

40. Dahlgren, E., Friberg, L.G., Johansson, S., Lindstrom, B., Oden, A., Samsioe, G., and Janson, P.O., Endometrial carcinoma: ovarian dysfunction—a risk factor in young women, *Eur. J. Obstet. Gynecol. Reprod. Biol.*, 41, 143, 1991.

41. Persson, I., Naessen, T., Adami, H.O., Bergstron, R., Lagrelius, A., Mollerstrom, G., Pettersson, B., and von Hamos, K., Reduced risk of hip fracture in women with endometrial cancer, *Int. J. Epidemiol.*, 21, 636, 1992.

42. Persson, I., Adami, H.O., McLaughlin, J.K., Naessen, T., and Fraumeni, J.F., Jr., Reduced risk of breast and endometrial cancer among women with hip fractures (Sweden), *Cancer Causes Control*, 5, 523, 1994.

43. Swanson, C.A., Potischman, N., Barrett, R.J., Berman, M.L., Mortel, R., Twiggs, L.B., Wilbanks, G.D., Hoover, R.N., and Brinton, L.A., Endometrial cancer risk in relation to serum lipids and lipoprotein levels, *Cancer Epidemiol. Biomarkers Prev.*, 3, 575, 1994.

44. Maatela, J., Aromaa, A., Salmi, T., Pohja, M., Vuento, M., and Gronroos, M., The risk of endometrial cancer in diabetic and hypertensive patients: a nationwide record-linkage study in Finland, *Ann. Chir. Gynaecol.*, 208, 20, 1994.

45. La Vecchia, C., Negri, E., Franceschi, S., D'Avanzo, B., and Boyle, P., A case-control study of diabetes mellitus and cancer risk, *Br. J. Cancer*, 70, 950, 1994.

46. Finkle, W.D., Greenland, S., Miettinen, O.S., and Ziel, H.K., Endometrial cancer risk after discontinuing use of unopposed conjugated estrogens (California, USA), *Cancer Causes Control*, 6, 99, 1995.

47. Rutqvist, L.E., Johansson, H., Signomklao, T., Johansson, U., Fornander, T., and Wilking, N., Adjuvant tamoxifen therapy for early stage breast cancer and second primary malignancies. Stockholm Breast Cancer Study Group, *J. Natl. Cancer Inst.*, 87, 645, 1995.

48. Cuenca, R.E., Giachino, J., Arredondo, M.A., Hempling, R., and Edge, S.B., Endometrial carcinoma associated with breast carcinoma: low incidence with tamoxifen use, *Cancer*, 77, 2058, 1996.

49. Potischman, N., Hoover, R.N., Brinton, L.A., Sitteri, P., Dorgan, J.F., Swanson, C.A., Berman, M.L., Mortel, R., Twiggs, L.B., Barrett, R.J., Wilbanks, G.D., Persky, V., and Lurain, J.R., Case-control study of endogenous steroid hormones and endometrial cancer, *J. Natl. Cancer Inst.*, 88, 1127, 1996.

50. Brinton, L.A., Barrett, R.J., Berman, M.L., Mortel, R., Twiggs, L.B., and Wilbanks, G.D., Cigarette smoking and the risk of endometrial cancer, *Am. J. Epidemiol.*, 137, 281, 1993.

51. Parazzini, F., La Vecchia, C., Bocciolone, L., and Franceschi, S., The epidemiology of endometrial cancer, *Gynecol. Oncol.*, 41, 1, 1991.

52. Folsom, A.R., Kaye, S.A., Potter, J.D., and Prineas, R.J., Association of incident carcinoma of the endometrium with body weight and fat distribution in older women: early findings of the Iowa Women's Health Study, *Cancer Res.*, 49, 6828, 1989.

53. Elwood, J.M., Cole, P., Rothman, K.J., and Kaplan, S.D., Epidemiology of endometrial cancer, *J. Natl. Cancer Inst.*, 59, 1055, 1977.

54. Henderson, B.E., Casagrande, J.T., Pike, M.C., Mack, T., and Rosario, I., The epidemiology of endometrial cancer in young women, *Br. J. Cancer*, 47, 749, 1983.

55. La Vecchia, C.A., Decarli, M., Fasoli, M., and Gentile, A., Nutrition and diet in the etiology of endometrial cancer, *Cancer*, 57, 1248, 1986.

56. Lew, E.A. and Garfinkel, L., Variations in mortality by weight among 750,000 men and women, *J. Chronic Dis.*, 32, 563, 1979.

57. Wynder, E.L., Escher, G.C., and Mantel, N., An epidemiological investigation of cancer of the endometrium, *Cancer*, 19, 489, 1966.

58. Shu, X.-O., Brinton, L.A., Zheng, W., Gao, Y.T., Fan, J., and Fraumeni, J.F., A population based case-control study of endometrial cancer in Shanghai, China, *Int. J. Cancer*, 49, 38, 1991.

59. Koumantaki, Y., Tzonou, A., Koumantakis, E., Kaklamani, E., Aravantinos, D., and Trichopoulos, D., A case-control study of cancer of the endometrium in Athens, *Int. J. Cancer*, 43, 795, 1989.

60. Schapira, D.V., Nutrition and cancer prevention, *Prim. Care*, 19, 481, 1992.

61. Lapidus, L., Helgesson, O., Merck, C., and Bjorntorp, P., Adipose tissue distribution and female carcinomas: a 12-year follow-up of participants in the population study of women in Goteborg, Sweden, *Int. J. Obesity*, 12, 361, 1988.

62. Levi, F., La Vecchia, C., Negri, E., Parazzini, F., and Franceschi, S., Body mass at different ages and subsequent endometrial cancer risk, *Int. J. Cancer*, 50, 567, 1992.

63. Olson, S.H., Trevisan, M., Marshall, J.R., Graham, S., Zielezny, M., Vena, J.E., Hellman, R., and Freudenheim, J.L., Body mass index, weight gain, and risk of endometrial cancer, *Nutr. Cancer*, 23, 141, 1995.

64. Swanson, C.A., Potischman, N., Wilbanks, G.D., Twiggs, L.B., Mortel, R., Berman, M.L., Barrett, R.J., Baumgartner, R.N., and Brinton, L.A., Relation of endometrial cancer risk to past and contemporary body size and body size distribution, *Cancer Epidemiol. Biomarkers Prev.*, 2, 321, 1993.

65. Levi, F., La Vecchia, C., Negri, E., and Franceschi, S., Selected physical activities and the risk of endometrial cancer, *Br. J. Cancer*, 67, 846, 1993.

66. Shu, X.O., Hatch, M.C., Zhang, W., Gao, Y.T., and Brinton, L.A., Physical activity and risk of endometrial cancer, *Epidemiology*, 4, 342, 1993.

67. La Vecchia, C., Nutritional factors and cancers of the breast, endometrium and ovary, *Eur. J. Cancer Clin. Oncol.*, 25, 1945, 1989.

68. Shu, X.O., Zheng, W., Potischman, N., Brinton, L.A., Hatch, M.C., Gao, Y.T., and Fraumeni, J.F., A population-based case-control study of dietary factors and endometrial cancer in Shanghai, People's Republic of China, *Am. J. Epidemiol.*, 137, 155, 1993.

69. Levi, F., Franceschi, S., Negri, E., and La Vecchia, C., Dietary factors and the risk of endometrial cancer, *Cancer*, 71, 3675, 1993.
70. Barbone, F., Austin, H., and Partridge, E.E., Diet and endometrial cancer: a case-control study, *Am. J. Epidemiol.*, 137, 393, 1993.
71. Potischman, N., Swanson, C.A., Brinton, L.A., McAdams, M., Barrett, R.J., Berman, M.L., Mortel, R., Twiggs, L.B., Wilbanks, G.D., and Hoover, R.N., Dietary associations in a case-control study of endometrial cancer, *Cancer Causes Control*, 4, 239, 1993.
72. de Meester, C. and Gerber, G.B., The role of cooked food mutagens as possible etiological agents in human cancer: a critical appraisal of recent epidemiological investigations, *Rev. Epidemiol. Sante Pub.*, 43, 147, 1995.
73. Zheng, W., Kushi, L.H., Potter, J.D., Sellers, T.A., Doyle, T.J., Bostick, R.M., and Folsom, A.R., Dietary intake of energy and animal foods and endometrial cancer incidence, *Am. J. Epidemiol.*, 142, 388, 1995.
74. Williams, R.R. and Horm, J.W., Association of cancer sites with tobacco and alcohol consumption and socioeconomic status of patients: interview study from the Third National Cancer Survey, *J. Natl. Cancer Inst.*, 58, 525, 1977.
75. Kato, I., Tominga, S., and Terao, C., Alcohol consumption and cancers of hormone-related organs in females, *Jpn. J. Clin. Oncol.*, 19, 202, 1989.
76. Webster, L.A., Weiss, N.S., and the Cancer and Steroid Hormone Study Group, Alcoholic beverage consumption and the risk of endometrial cancer, *Int. J. Epidemiol.*, 18, 786, 1989.
77. Swanson, C.A., Wilbanks, G.D., Twiggs, L.B., Mortel, R., Berman, M.L., Barrett, R.J., and Brinton, L.A., Moderate alcohol consumption and the risk of endometrial cancer, *Epidemiology*, 4, 530, 1993.
78. Armstrong, B.K., Brown, J.B., Clarke, H.T., Crooke, D.K., Hahnel, R., Masarei, J.R., and Ratajezak, T., Diet and reproductive hormones: a study of vegetarian and nonvegetarian postmenopausal women, *J. Natl. Cancer Inst.*, 67, 761, 1981.
79. Cauley, J.A., Gutaj, J.P., Kuller, L.H., LeDonne, D., and Powell, J.G., The epidemiology of serum sex hormones in postmenopausal women, *Am. J. Epidemiol.*, 129, 1120, 1989.
80. Gapstur, S.M., Potter, J.D., Sellars, T.A., Kushi, L.H., and Folsom, A.R., Alcohol consumption and postmenopausal endometrial cancer: results from the Iowa Women's Health Study, *Cancer Causes Control*, 4, 323, 1993.
81. Hill, H.A. and Austin, H., Nutrition and endometrial cancer, *Cancer Causes Control*, 7, 19, 1996.

CHAPTER 6

NUTRITION AND COLON CANCER IN WOMEN

CONTENTS

I. GENERAL PATHOLOGY AND STATISTICS

Colorectal cancer accounts for about 11% of all newly diagnosed cancers in women and 10% of all cancer-related deaths;[1] 98% of all cancers in the large intestine are adenocarcinomas. The peak incidence for colorectal carcinoma is age 60–70. With lesions in the rectum, the male-to-female ratio is 2:1; for more proximal tumors, there are some gender differences which will be discussed in a later section.

About 25% of carcinomas are generally located in the cecum or ascending colon and a similar proportion in the rectum and distal sigmoid; 25% are located in the descending colon and proximal sigmoid. The remainder are scattered elsewhere. Tumors in the proximal colon tend to grow as polypoid, fungating masses that extend along one wall. Obstruction is uncommon. When carcinomas in the distal colon are discovered, they tend to be annular, encircling lesions that produce so-called napkin-ring constrictions of the bowel. The lumen is usually markedly narrowed.

The microscopic characteristics of right-sided and left-sided colonic adenocarcinomas are similar. Differentiation may range from well differentiated to undifferentiated with frankly anaplastic lesions. Invasive tumor incites a strong desmoplastic stromal response, leading to the characteristic firm, hard consistency of most colonic carcinomas.[2] Colorectal cancers may remain asymptomatic for years.

Colorectal tumors spread by direct extension into adjacent structures and by metastasis through the lymphatics and blood vessels. The favored sites of metastatic spread are the regional lymph nodes, liver, lungs, and bones.

The single most important prognostic indicator of colorectal carcinoma is the extent of the tumor at the time of diagnosis. The Astler-Coller staging system[3,5] for colorectal carcinoma is a modification of the Dukes and Kirklin classification.[4] A patient with an Astler-Coller A lesion has a virtual 100% chance for 5-year survival after resection, falling to 67% for a B1 lesion, 54% for a B2 lesion, 43% for a C1 lesion, and 23% for a C2 lesion. The challenge is to discover these neoplasms when curative resection is possible. The disease has usually spread beyond the range of curative surgery in 25–30% of patients. The staging for colorectal neoplasms is shown in Table 6.1.[3,5]

II. POPULATION GENETICS AND MARKERS FOR RISK

A. Familial Adenomatous Polyposis

Colorectal cancer includes both hereditary and nonhereditary types. Hereditary colorectal cancer with an autosomal dominant mode of inheritance includes familial adenomatous polyposis (FAP) with numerous colonic polyps and also an even rarer syndrome that includes the adenomatosis of Gardner syndrome.[6] FAP is prototypic of the polyposis-related colorectal cancer syndromes, occurring with a frequency of 1 per 5000 or 1 per 10,000 live births, and it accounts for less than 1% of colorectal cancers in adult life.[6] Penetrance of FAP has been estimated to be 80–100%.[6] The gene involved in FAP is the

Table 6.1   Staging for Colorectal Neoplasms

Tumor Stage	Histologic Features of the Neoplasm
A	Limited to mucosa
B1	Extending into muscularis propria but not penetrating through it; uninvolved nodes
B2	Penetrating through muscularis propria; uninvolved nodes
C1	Extending into muscularis propria but not penetrating through it; involved nodes
C2	Penetrating through muscularis propria; involved nodes
D	Distant metastatic spread

From Astler, V.B. and Coller, F.A., *Ann. Surg.*, 139, 846, 1954. With permission.

APC (adenomatous polyposis coli) gene, which mapped to chromosome 5q21.[6] The identification of the *APC* gene was facilitated by recognition of an interstitial deletion of 5q in a patient with adenomatous polyposis of Gardner syndrome and mental retardation.[7,8] The cumulative incidence of FAP in these patients approaches 100% by age 55, and large bowel carcinoma develops about 20 years earlier than in the general population. In Gardner syndrome, patients have extraintestinal lesions as well, osteomas, epidermal inclusion cysts, cutaneous fibromas, abnormal dentition, and dentigerous cysts.[6] Turcot syndrome is a rare autosomal recessive syndrome associated with adenomatous polyposis of the large intestine, astrocytomas of the central nervous system, and basal cell carcinomas of the skin.[9] Numerous point and frameshift mutations of the *APC* gene have been identified, but it has been suggested that the site of the mutation, such as a deletion in codon 1309 in exon 15, may be an unfavorable prognostic marker of severity of neoplastic disease.[6]

B. Hereditary Nonpolyposis Colon Cancer

Another common type of hereditary colon cancer is hereditary nonpolyposis colorectal cancer (HNPCC), which occurs without multiple polyps. This is also transmitted by an autosomal dominant form of inheritance, is more common than FAP, and may actually account for 5–10% of the colorectal cancer in the United States. HNPCC includes two syndromes: Lynch syndrome I, which is hereditary site-specific colon cancer, and Lynch syndrome II, the cancer family syndrome. In Lynch syndrome I, the increased risk of colorectal cancer is expressed 15–20 years earlier than in the general population and occurs in the absence of polyposis. In this syndrome, two-thirds of the lesions occur in the proximal or right half of the colon.[6] HNPCC and FAP make up the majority of hereditary colorectal cancers, with the nonhereditary type being referred to as sporadic colon cancer, which develops in patients without strong family histories.

C. Loss of Heterozygosity

Previous analysis of many tumors from patients with both FAP and sporadic colon cancer for loss of heterozygosity (LOH) on chromosomes 5q, 8p, 17p, 18q, and 22q and mutation of the A*PC* gene, *p53*, and K-*ras* genes has shown that there is an adenoma–carcinoma sequence that occurs in most colorectal cancer, and it starts with the development of an adenoma.[10] In 1988, the landmark paper describing the accumulation of molecular genetic alterations during the adenoma–carcinoma sequence was first published by Vogelstein et al.[11] This study showed the prevalence of allelic deletions of 5q, 18q, and 17p in adenomas and cancers and established the favored sequence of events. The resulting model of these accumulated changes in oncogenes has been refined over time, and this model has become the paradigm for the molecular events seen in development of neoplasia.[12] The mechanism involves the accumulation of genetic changes in multiple tumor suppressor genes as follows:[10, 12] inactivation of the *APC* gene by two mutations is involved in the development of mild to moderate adenoma; LOH of the *APC* gene is associated with further development to carcinoma; mutation and LOH of the *p53* gene is involved in the conversion of adenoma to early carcinoma; LOH on 8p, 19q, and 22q is involved in the progression of early carcinoma to advanced carcinoma; and K-*ras* mutation affects the growth of tumors. The loci on 8p and 18q have subsequently been identified as the *myc* and *DCC* (deleted in colon cancer) genes, respectively.[10] It is currently believed that the development of most sporadic colon tumors follows this molecular sequence. However, few genetic changes, such as LOH and *APC* mutation, were found in tumors from HNPCC patients.[10] These findings led to the idea that tumors from HNPCC patients had different mechanisms than those seen in FAP and sporadic colon cancer patients.

D. Microsatellite Instability

It has now been determined that microsatellite instability, or replication error, is a characteristic of tumors in HNPCC. A mutated genetic locus (hMSH2) has been mapped to chromosome 2p15-16, and this is associated with about 60% of the familial colon cancer of HNPCC.[13–15] Preliminary studies have shown this to be the locus of a mismatch repair gene that gives rise to alterations in short, repeated sequences of DNA, which confers on these cells a mutator phenotype, enhancing the mutability of the entire human genome.[13–16] A second mismatch repair gene was subsequently identified on chromosome 3q21 (hMLH1) which, when mutated, may account for another 30% of cases of HNPCC.[6] These two genes encode enzymes that ensure the integrity of the DNA repair pathway, and when mutated, mismatch repair is impaired in these cancer cells.

More recently, it has been shown that there are also some kindreds in Utah with an excess of colorectal cancer cases that do not meet the strict criteria for HNPCC, nor do they demonstrate linkage to the genes in the adenoma–carcinoma sequence of Fearon and Vogelstein[12] or any of the mismatch repair genes hMSH2, hMLH1, hPMS1, and hPMS2.[17] DiVinci et al.[18] have provided convincing evidence implicating chromosome 1p deletions in the early development of colorectal tumors. The search is currently on for a chromosome 1p tumor suppressor gene, which may also play an important role in colorectal carcinogenesis.

In summary, the genetics of colorectal cancer has been better delineated than for any other common cancer. However, the myriad genetic defects seen in the different familial and sporadic forms of this cancer still account for only 10–15% of all cases of colorectal cancer. Much work clearly still remains in understanding the genesis of these common tumors. All of the genetic work has been done on kindreds displaying a high incidence of these cancers and, as such, involved both men and women. Although there appear to be significant differences in the biology of colorectal cancer between men and women, there is no reason at this time to believe that there are any inherent genetic differences in the molecular development of tumors in men and women. Therefore, all of the above-described genetic pathways can be assumed to be similar for all colon cancer, regardless of gender.

III. GENERAL EPIDEMIOLOGY OF COLON CANCER IN WOMEN

A. Gender Differences

Colorectal cancer is the second most common cancer in women after breast cancer, and the age-adjusted colonic cancer incidence per 100,000 in the United States for 1985–89 was 34% higher for males than for females.[6] The male predominance for rectal cancer was even more pronounced at 73%. During the years 1973–85, the incidence in males increased 19%, and during 1985–89, it rose 6%,[6] whereas for females during the same time periods, it rose 9% and then declined by 10%, respectively. The distribution of the colonic neoplasms is also sex-related. Right-sided colon cancer includes cecum, ascending colon, hepatic flexure, and transverse colon, whereas left-sided would include the splenic flexure, descending colon, sigmoid, rectosigmoid, and rectum. Male colon cancers in those above age 65 tend to be predominantly on the left side, including the rectum, and female colon cancers tend to predominate in all subsites in the colon except the rectum at ages below 65.[19] Interestingly, incidence rates in men and women cross around the age of menopause, with male rates, previously lower, subsequently exceeding female rates.[20] In 1969, Fraumeni et al.[21] reported that there was an elevated risk of colon cancer in nuns, in addition to breast cancer. This and other sex and age differences led McMichael and Potter in 1980[20] to postulate that the hormonal milieu associated with pregnancy probably resulted in lower risk for colon cancer in women. They also further postulated that exogenous hormone use could lower the risk of colon cancer in women.

B. Reproductive Factors

Initial data on reproductive factors such as parity/age at first birth seemed to indicate that early pregnancy conferred protection against colon cancer in women,[22-24] but further studies showed no association.[25] Thus, the reproductive history is not consistent or uncomplicated. However, a very recent investigation from the Nurses' Health Study cohort by Martinez et al.[26] explored the roles of reproductive factors and oral contraceptive use in the etiology of colorectal cancer. They examined 501 incident cases of colorectal cancer during 12 years of follow-up in this cohort.[26] In a multivariate analysis, the relative risk of colorectal cancer among women who experienced late menarche at age 14 or older was 0.83 compared with women who had menarche at age 13. For those whose menarche occurred under age 12, the relative risk was 1.22. For first pregnancy occurring over age 30, the relative risk was 1.57 compared with women whose first pregnancy occurred before age 24.[26] There were no significant associations with parity or age at menopause. Women who were users of oral contraceptives for a period of over 96 months had a 40% lower risk of developing colorectal cancer.[26] The data from this prospective study indicate that the use of oral contraceptives may reduce the risk of colorectal cancer, although paradoxically, women who postpone first pregnancy may be at higher risk.[26]

C. Hormone Replacement Therapy

Exogenous hormone use appears to have emerged as a more straightforward association. Potter and McMichael[23] initially observed that oral contraceptive use was associated with lower risk, a finding that has not been supported in more recent investigations.[27] In fact, one study in China[28] reported that there is an increased risk of colon cancer in Chinese females with hormone replacement therapy (HRT). One of the more recent studies by Risch and Howe[29] was a record linkage cohort study of menopausal hormone use and colorectal cancer in Saskatchewan. These authors[29] found that of 230 first primary cases of colorectal cancer occurring, women who took estrogens had a nonsignificant elevated risk of colon cancer in general and cancer of the distal colon in particular (relative risk of 1.51). In this study, women who took oral contraceptives had a significantly increased risk (relative risk = 2.12) for cancer of the proximal colon, although the authors state that this could also have occurred by chance.[29] They summarized that their study did not support the hypothesis that use of HRT is associated with risk of colorectal cancer. However, a number of recent studies of HRT have found that there is a lower risk associated with HRT.[30, 31]

Calle et al.[30] used a large cohort of women from the American Cancer Society's Cancer Prevention Study-II to assess the relationship between ever use of HRT and risk of fatal colon cancer. They found that the ever use of HRT was significantly associated with decreased risk of fatal colon cancer, with a relative risk of 0.71. The reduction in risk was strongest among current users (relative risk = 0.55).[30] These associations were not changed by controlling for other risk factors. Following Calle et al.'s publication by a few months, Newcomb and Storer[31] reported their evaluation of postmenopausal hormone use in a population-based case-control study of large-bowel cancer among Wisconsin women. This study used 694 case subjects and 1622 randomly selected community control subjects and analyzed HRT use and family and medical history in telephone interviews.[31] Their results indicated that recent users of HRT had a relative risk for colon cancer of 0.54 and a relative risk for rectal cancer of 0.91, compared with women who had never used HRT.[31] Interestingly, the effect of HRT was more pronounced in those women judged to be at lower absolute risk of colon cancer, i.e., those with lean body mass.[31] These associations were observed among users of both estrogen alone and the combined estrogen and progestin preparations. Finally, in the most recent study published, Potter et al.[32] undertook a case-control study in Minnesota women to determine if HRT was associated with lower risk of adenomatous polyps. This case-control study utilized cases from the Minnesota Cancer Prevention Research Unit and compared them with two control groups: women without polyps at colonoscopy and women controls selected from the general community.[32] Significant findings were that the odds ratios for the use of HRT for less than 5 years compared to never use were 0.52 vs. colonoscopy controls and 0.74 vs. community controls for postmenopausal women. For 5 years of use or greater, the corresponding odds ratios for the two control groups were 0.39 and 0.61. Thus, in the most recent studies published, there is emerging a clear risk-lowering effect of HRT in postmenopausal women, both for colorectal cancer and for adenomatous polyps.

D. Cigarette Smoking

Another risk factor associated with colorectal adenoma and colorectal cancer among women in the United States is cigarette smoking.[33] Although a positive correlation between smoking and colorectal cancer had previously been reported for men, it had not previously been considered a risk factor for women until Giovanucci et al.[33] examined the association between smoking and colorectal cancer in women. Consistent with the other studies of smoking and risk of colorectal cancer in women,[33] only a weak, statistically nonsignificant association between smoking and colon cancer in women was noted in the first report from the Nurses' Health Study.[34] In the latest report from the Nurses' Health Study,[33] the purpose was to assess the association between smoking and colorectal cancer in women and also to estimate the minimum induction period between the onset of smoking and cancer diagnosis. The authors documented 586 new cases of colorectal cancer from 1976 to 1990 and 564 cases of adenoma among 12,143 women.[33] They then assessed the relative risk associated with pack-years of smoking for small adenoma, larger adenoma (greater than 1 cm), and for colorectal cancer. The risk for each stage in the carcinoma sequence was related to dose of cigarette smoking in terms of pack-years. The amount of smoking in the previous 20 years was only related to risk for small adenomas (relative risk = 1.45) and not large adenomas (relative risk = 1.31). However, as smoking went back more than 20 years in the past, pack-years were related to risk for large adenomas (relative risk = 1.29) and not for small adenomas (relative risk = 1.11). Cigarette smoking was not related to colorectal cancer until 35 years after smoking was initiated in that for women who had smoked more than ten cigarettes per day for 35–39 years past, the relative risk for cancer was 1.47, progressing to 1.63 after 40–44 years and 2.00 after 45 years.[33] These authors concluded that because the minimum induction period for colorectal cancer appears to be at least 35 years, the association between smoking and colorectal cancer in women is just now showing up. In a recent review of tobacco, colorectal cancer, and adenomas by this same group,[35] the authors actually postulate that the increasing male-to-female mortality ratio from colorectal cancer over the latter half of this century in the United States may have been a result of greater tobacco use by men earlier in this century and go on to state that they believe that approximately 20% of large-bowel cancers are attributable to smoking. This does not bode well for the incidence of large-bowel cancers in women in the foreseeable future based on current estimates of a 35-year induction period for these tumors.[33]

E. Nonsteroidal Anti-Inflammatory Drugs

Recent epidemiological studies have provided increasingly convincing evidence for a role of regular nonsteroidal anti-inflammatory drug (NSAID) use and decreased risk for colorectal cancer.[36] Eight previous studies have specifically examined the relationship between regular NSAID use and colorectal cancer in women with mixed results, but generally there was a trend for reduction in risk with NSAID use.[36] Reeves et al.[36] have recently reported on the use of NSAIDs and protection against colorectal cancer in an ongoing population-based case-control study in Wisconsin women; 184 cases and 293 controls were assessed on their regular use of NSAIDs, which was defined as usage at least twice weekly for 12 months or longer. After adjustment of the data for age, controls were more likely than cases to report regular NSAID use (38% vs. 27%). Following adjustment for age, prior sigmoidoscopy, family history of colorectal cancer, and body mass index, women who used NSAIDs regularly were less likely to be diagnosed with colorectal cancer than were women who did not use NSAIDs (odds ratio = 0.65, no consistent trend with duration of use). When the type of NSAID was studied, nonaspirin compounds appeared to confer greater protection compared to nonusers than did aspirin (odds ratio = 0.43 vs. 0.79 for aspirin). These data support the idea that NSAID use is protective against colorectal cancer in women and also that aspirin may not be the best choice of NSAID.

We have been careful in our discussion of colorectal cancer epidemiology and risk factors to emphasize only those data specific to women. There are, of course, large numbers of studies on men alone, as well as on men and women combined, and we have attempted to limit our discussion to those studies pertinent to women alone, wherever possible.

IV. PHYSICAL ACTIVITY AND INDICATORS OF GENERAL NUTRITION

Low levels of physical activity and high levels of energy intake and body mass have all been directly associated with colon cancer in both men and women. A number of studies have shown consistently that being physically active has been associated with a lower risk of colon cancer, but how this all related to high energy intake and greater body mass has not been consistent.[37] Slattery and colleagues[37] have attempted to determine how physical activity interacted with other components of energy balance, such as energy intake and body mass, in determining colon cancer risk in both men and women. For both men and women, lack of lifetime vigorous leisure-time activity was associated with increased risk of colon cancer, with an odds ratio of 1.63 for men and 1.59 for women[37] when comparing the lowest to the highest level of activity. High levels of energy intake were also associated with increased colon cancer risk in both men and women, with odds ratios of 1.74 and 1.70, respectively. A large body mass index was more associated with risk in men than in women, with odds ratios of 1.94 and 1.45, respectively. For those who had all three risk factors—low physical activity, high energy intake, and large body mass—the odds ratio was 3.35 and was consistent between both men and women. However, in the presence of higher physical activity, a high energy intake and large body mass only nonsignificantly increased colon cancer risk in both sexes. Additionally, there was some evidence that men may be at higher risk than women in the presence of an unfavorable energy balance.[37]

Along a similar theme, frequency of eating and risk of colorectal cancer has been studied in women. Generally, food intake patterns have been infrequently studied with regard to colon cancer risk. A recent study of Wisconsin women with a new diagnosis of cancer of the colon or rectum during 1990–91 was identified from the statewide cancer registry.[38] Community control subjects were used, and meal and snack frequency was obtained on a subset of cases and controls. Compared with women consuming three or four meals daily, women who consumed only one or two meals daily had a relative risk of only 0.57 for colorectal cancer,[38] whereas snack frequency and meals plus snacks were not associated with cancer risk in this population. These data are consistent with several other studies that have evaluated meal frequency and found that those who eat more often usually have an elevated risk of colorectal cancer.[38] However, the authors urge caution in the interpretation of their results, in that they suggest that the nutrient composition of the meals and snacks may be more relevant than the association of meal frequency with more frequent release of colon cancer–promoting bile acids.

V. DIETARY FAT, RED MEAT, AND HETEROCYCLIC AMINES

The hypothesis that dietary meat and/or fat increases risk of colon cancer has been the predominant hypothesis relevant to colon carcinogenesis for the past 20 years. The role of dietary fat and meat consumption has been extensively reviewed elsewhere by Potter et al.[39] These authors found that 13 of 24 epidemiologic studies analyzed found a direct association between meat consumption and colon cancer, and 10 of 18 studies found a direct association between fat and colon cancer. Although some of these studies may have had women as participants, the most notable studies of dietary fat and colon cancer risk in women are the Nurses' Health Study[40] and the Iowa Women's Health Study.[41] These were both large prospective studies limited to women who used the same dietary assessment questionnaire. In the Nurses' Health Study, the authors reported a direct association between the intake of fat and meat and the risk for colorectal cancer, whereas the Iowa Women's Health Study reported a null association. In the Nurses' Health Study, after adjustment for total energy intake, animal fat was positively associated with the risk of colon cancer, with the relative risk for the highest compared with the lowest quintile at 1.89. The relative risk for women who ate beef, pork, or lamb as a main dish every day was 2.49.[40] However, in the Iowa Women's Health Study, there was no association found.[41] But, as pointed out by Willett et al.,[40,42] the interpretation of many studies of fat, meat, and colon cancer is hampered by the common finding of a direct association between total energy intake and risk (Table 6.2).

The most recent twist on the meat/colon cancer connection is that of the heterocyclic amines (HCAs) present in well-cooked meat. Proponents of this hypothesis linking meat and colon cancer make the case that it is not the meat per se that increases risk, but that it is the generation of carcinogenic HCA compounds during the high-temperature cooking of meat that is the culprit. Although there are no separate reports of colon cancer in women linked to

Table 6.2   Studies of Nutrients and Colorectal Cancer Risk in Women

Nutrient	Type of Study[a]	Association with Risk[b]	Reference
Meat	Review[c]	Direct, 13 of 24 studies	39
Fat intake	Review[c]	Direct, 10 of 18 studies	39
Meat, fat	NHS	Direct, RR = 2.49	40
	IWHS	No association	41
Calcium	NHS	No association	40
	IWHS	Decreased, nonsignificant	45
	Case-control[c]	Decreased, OR = 0.50[d]	46
	Case-control	Decreased, OR = 0.56	47
Vitamin D	NHS	No significant association	40
	IWHS	Inverse, nonsignificant	45
Dairy foods	Case-control[c]	Inverse, OR = 0.53[d]	46
	Case-control	Decreased, RR = 0.59	47
Calcium, vitamin D, dairy foods	Prospective cohort[c]	No association with colorectal adenomas[d]	48
Vitamin E	IWHS	Inverse, RR = 0.32	49
	NHS	No association	44
	Clinical trial[c]	Inverse, nonsignificant[d]	51
Vitamin A	Case-control	No association	55
	Case-control	Inverse, RR = 0.7	56
	Prospective	No association	58
Beta-carotene	Prospective	No association	59
Fiber from vegetables	Case-control	Inverse	47, 65
Fiber	Case-control	Direct, in older women	55
Fruits, vegetables	IWHS	Inverse, RR = 0.73	68
Fiber from fruits and vegetables	NHS	No association	40
Vegetables	Mortality rate study among vegetarians	Reduced death rate for women[d]	69
Sucrose	Case-control[c]	Direct, RR = 1.13[d]	73
	IWHS	Direct, RR = 2.0	41
Folate	NHS	Inverse, RR = 0.66	74
Alcohol	NHS	Direct, RR = 1.84	74

[a] IWHS = Iowa Women's Health Study, prospective cohort study. NHS = Nurses' Health Study, prospective cohort.
[b] RR = relative risk; OR = odds ratio.
[c] Studies included both men and women.
[d] Outcome reported for women only.

HCAs, a case-control study in Stockholm examined the associations between methods of cooking meats and colorectal cancer. The highest relative risks were for fried meat with a heavily browned meat surface, with a relative risk for colon cancer of 2.8 and for rectum cancer of 6.0.[43] These data support the findings of Willett et al.[40] for red meat intake.

VI. DAIRY FOODS, CALCIUM, AND VITAMIN D

The epidemiologic literature on calcium and colon cancer is extensive by now (Table 6.2), and inverse associations have been more frequently found, although the data are still inconsistent (for an excellent review, see Bostick[44]). However, one of the studies which demonstrated no association was the Nurses' Health Study,[40] which used the same food frequency questionnaire as the Iowa Women's Health Study,[45] although there was seen in the latter a nonsignificant decrease in risk after multivariate adjustment (relative risk of 0.68). However, in a Utah study that included men and women, Slattery et al.[46] reported a halving of colon cancer risk for both men and women (adjusted odds ratio = 0.50 for females) for those in the highest quartile of calcium intake. Kune et al.,[47] in an Australian case-control study, had found an odds ratio of 0.56 for women with the highest calcium intake.

There have only been six epidemiologic studies to date that investigated the association of vitamin D and colon cancer,[44] and only four have reported an inverse association. Again, the only studies limited to women were the Nurses' Health Study,[40] which reported no significant association with no relative risk/odds ratio given, and the Iowa Women's Health Study,[45] which reported a suggested inverse association with a nonsignificant relative risk of 0.73. None of the other studies separated associations by gender if they did include both males and females.

Milk product intake has also been rather extensively studied in relation to risk for colorectal cancer. However, there was only one study that reported a strong association between intake of milk products and colon cancer risk, and that was a study in Utah[46] which focused specifically on calcium and milk in relation to colon cancer. Relatively high milk intake was significantly associated with reduction in risk in both men and women, where the adjusted odds ratios were 0.44 and 0.53, respectively. Kune et al.[47] in the Melbourne study reported a significant reduction in risk for women only (relative risk = 0.59). Otherwise, in the majority of studies, no major patterns have emerged. As a final note, Kampman et al.[48] examined calcium, vitamin D, dairy foods, and the occurrence of colorectal adenomas among men and women in two prospective studies. These authors concluded that colorectal adenoma was related to neither calcium intake nor to milk consumption, whereas vitamin D from supplement use, but not from diet, was slightly but not significantly inversely associated with risk in women only.

VII. ANTIOXIDANT VITAMINS

Antioxidant micronutrients, which for the purposes of our discussion will include vitamin E, vitamin C, the carotenoids and vitamin A, and selenium, defend the body against free radicals and reactive oxygen molecules and have been implicated in the dietary prevention of cancer, especially colorectal cancer (Table 6.2). Relatively few epidemiological studies have addressed dietary antioxidant intake and the risk of colon cancer, especially in women. Bostick et al.[49] performed a prospective cohort study in women to address the association of colon cancer with vitamin E intake and selenium supplement use in a well-defined population of postmenopausal women from the Iowa Women's Health Study. The mailed questionnaire was identical to the one used by the 1984 Nurses' Health Study.[50] The food frequency questionnaire covered usual food intake and vitamin and mineral supplement use. The specific information solicited on vitamin and mineral supplement use included the dose per day of specific nutrient supplements, the name of the multivitamin/mineral pills used, and the number of such pills taken per week.[49] The amount of each antioxidant micronutrient taken was calculated from a nutrient database. After adjustment for age, the total vitamin E intake was found to be inversely associated with the risk of colon cancer in women,[49] with a relative risk for the highest quintile compared to the lowest of 0.32. There was no change when further adjusted for total energy intake and other risk factors.[49] There was also a decreasing effect of vitamin E with advancing age. The relative risks for the age groups 55–59, 60–64, and 65–69 years of age were 0.16, 0.37, and 0.93, respectively.[49] There were no significant effects of supplemental intakes of vitamins A and C, beta-carotene, or selenium in this population of postmenopausal women. In the only other prospective cohort study in women (Nurses' Health Study), vitamin E intake and colon cancer were not associated.[44]

In a clinical trial of antioxidant vitamin supplementation to prevent colorectal adenoma,[51] both male and female adenoma patients received either placebo, 25 mg/day beta-carotene, 1 g vitamin C plus 400 mg vitamin E per day, or the combination of both beta-carotene and vitamins C and E. The primary endpoint for analysis was the incidence of new colorectal adenomas. There was no evidence that either beta-carotene or vitamins C and E reduced the incidence of adenomas, with the relative risk being 1.01 for beta-carotene and 1.08 for the vitamins. However, when the data were separated by sex, there was a lowering of the relative risk for females taking vitamins C and E down to 0.81, although this did not appear to be significant. However, there were only about 20% women in this trial, so perhaps the authors should have included more women and maybe a significant effect could have been found. In general, a meta-analysis of five prospective, nested case-control studies showed that high serum or plasma levels of alpha-tocopherol were associated with a small decrease in the subsequent risk for development of colorectal cancer,[52] but these studies contained both sexes with no separate odds ratios given by sex. For the five studies analyzed, the matched odds ratio for the highest quartile of serum alpha-tocopherol concentration compared with the lowest was 0.6 and was 0.7 after adjustment for serum cholesterol level.[52] These results suggest that serum alpha-tocopherol concentration may be inversely related to risk of colorectal cancer.

A very recent double-blind, placebo-controlled clinical study of 1312 patients with a history of basal or squamous cell carcinomas of the skin found, as a secondary endpoint, that selenium supplementation of 200 μg selenium per day reduced the incidence of colorectal cancer in this population.[53] This trial contained both men and women, and there was no breakdown of separate effects for women. However, a previous report[54] by this group has shown that fasting plasma selenium concentrations may be an important risk factor for colorectal adenomas. Patients with fasting plasma selenium concentrations below the median (<128 μg/l) were significantly more likely (3.5 times) to have one or more adenomatous polyps per patient.[54] Again, these data demonstrated no breakdown by gender.

Relatively few studies have examined vitamin A intake and colon cancer. In a large case-control study in Australia, Potter and McMichael[55] did not observe a substantial protective effect for either preformed vitamin A or carotenoids in either men or women for either colon or rectal cancer. Lyon et al.[56] in a Utah case-control study observed a small protective effect for intake of total vitamin A in women only (relative risk = 0.7). In a subsequent Utah study,[57] a protective effect was seen in both men and women (relative risk = 0.5) for higher intake of beta-carotene. In two prospective studies of vitamin A and carotenoid intake, no effect was seen in a California study by Paganini-Hill et al.,[58] but Heilbrun et al.[59] did observe a modest protective effect among men, but not in women, of a higher intake of beta-carotene. A very recent study examined whether the intakes of the main dietary carotenoids or vitamins A, C, or E were associated with the prevalence of colorectal adenomas among male and female patients who were members of a health plan in Los Angeles and who had undergone sigmoidoscopy.[60] Although the study contained 33% women participants, the data were pooled and not separated as to gender. In general, the data provided only modest support for the hypothesis that beta-carotene is protective against the development of colorectal adenomatous polyps.[60]

VIII. FIBER, FRUITS, AND VEGETABLES

A large body of evidence from both epidemiological and experimental studies has suggested that colon cancer risk can be reduced by a high intake of dietary fiber or other components associated with a diet high in vegetables, grains, or fruit (Table 6.2).[61–63] A meta-analysis of the large body of epidemiological research on dietary fiber and vegetables and the risk of colorectal cancer was undertaken, and the data revealed that the majority of the studies gave support for a protective effect associated with fiber-rich diets.[63] An odds ratio of 0.57 was obtained when the highest and lowest quintiles of intake were compared. The risk estimates for vegetables were only 0.48, thus underscoring the difficulty of separating out the effects of vegetables from a fiber-rich diet in the protection against colon cancer. However, only three[47,64,65] of the case-control studies assessed showed separate effects for males and females, and there was a significant protective effect of high-fiber vegetables in only two of them.[47,65] In contrast, Potter and McMichael[55] reported a study in which there was a significant lack of a protective effect of fiber, specifically an excess risk associated with cereal fiber in older women.

A more recent examination of the effect of dietary fiber on colonic diacylglycerols (DAGs) in women[66] showed that all sources of dietary fiber increased the amount of fecal fat excreted, which is associated with decreased cancer risk. Wheat bran decreased the concentrations of total DAGs, compounds which are thought to enhance excess colonic cell proliferation and increase risk for colon cancer. A recent study[67] which also separated by gender the examination of the effects of diet on risk of colorectal adenomas demonstrated that intake of fruit and fiber derived from fruits and vegetables was inversely related to adenomas in women (P for trend = 0.28 and 0.12, respectively). Total fat also showed a positive association in women, with an odds ratio of 2.69 for a comparison between the highest and lowest quintiles.[67] Interestingly, the risks for men were generally similar but were not statistically significant.

The only prospective study to report combined fruit and vegetable findings in relation to colon cancer incidence was the Iowa Women's Health Study.[68] These authors found a relative risk of 0.73 for combined vegetable and fruit intake and 0.68 for garlic. The Nurses' Health Study analyzed fiber intake from fruits and vegetables and found no significant associations.[40] There have not been any reports to date of clinical trials of vegetable and fruit consumption and risk of colon cancer.[44] Interestingly, in Germany, a study[69] assessed mortality and morbidity risks for colon cancer as related to nutritional status of moderate and strict vegetarians. Compared with national mortality rates, the observed deaths from colon cancer were reduced in men and women (standard mortality ratio for women = 77.9).

IX. OTHER DIETARY FACTORS

Sucrose intake has been examined in relation to colon cancer risk in a number of studies.[44] To date, 13 epidemiologic studies have investigated the association of sucrose consumption and colon cancer, with an increased risk seen in 11 of them, but these were statistically significant in only 4.[41,70–72] Only one of these[73] gave a separate odds ratio/relative risk for women, and that was only 1.13. In the only prospective study of sucrose and colon cancer, the Iowa Women's Health Study[41] reported a relative risk of 2.0 for colon cancer in women consuming high intakes of sucrose and sucrose-containing foods.[41]

The Nurses' Health Study was also used to assess the dietary intake of folate, methionine, and alcohol on the risk for colorectal adenoma.[74] With the major sources of folate being fruits and vegetables, it seemed appropriate to investigate the actual intake of folate in this major prospective cohort. Results indicated that high dietary folate was inversely associated with risk of colorectal adenoma in women, with a relative risk of 0.66 between high and low quintiles of intake.[74] Also studied in this investigation was the effect of alcohol consumption in these women. Relative to nondrinkers, women who consumed more than 30 g of alcohol per day (about two drinks) had an elevated risk of adenoma, with a relative risk of 1.84.[74] The authors state that these data support efforts to increase dietary folate in subpopulations who have low intakes of this nutrient.[74] A few other studies of alcohol and colon cancer in women have generally yielded results that have demonstrated little association between alcohol consumption and colorectal cancer or polyps (Table 6.2) (for review, see Potter et al.[39]).

X. GENERAL CONCLUSIONS, SUMMARY, AND IMPLICATIONS

The genetics of colorectal cancer, although well defined and delineated as to where and when specific mutations participate in the carcinogenesis process, can account for only about 10–15% of cancers. That leaves over 85% which are considered to be nonfamilial and which may have a significant dietary etiology in both men and women.

However, the hormonal environment for women is quite different from that of men, and as such, we see an intriguing impact of female reproductive factors on colorectal cancer in women. It would appear that some of the factors which influence risk for breast cancer, such as early pregnancy and later menarche, may also decrease risk for colon cancer in women. However, exogenous hormone use, either as oral contraceptives or estrogen replacement therapy, has been seen in some studies to be protective and in others as risk-enhancing. Interestingly, the most recent studies published appear to definitely support the hypothesis that HRT in postmenopausal women lowers their risk of colorectal cancer.

Long-term use of tobacco and alcohol consumption have been linked to many cancers, among them colorectal cancer. The long induction period for colorectal cancer associated with tobacco use has allowed the connection in women to finally emerge. As for alcoholic beverage consumption, a small number of studies have been done in women and have not demonstrated strong associations between alcohol and colorectal cancer or polyps, although the Nurses' Health Study cohort has shown an elevated risk. NSAID use in women has been shown to somewhat reduce colorectal cancer risk, with nonaspirin compounds appearing to confer greater protection.

The scientific literature has been absolutely inundated during the past 20 years with studies of dietary factors and risk for colorectal cancer. However, only a small number of these studies have separated the results by gender, and only a very few of them have examined the influence of dietary intake in women alone. In general, for both males and females, there is increased risk associated with a large body mass index, low levels of physical activity, and high energy intake.

When examining the role of specific nutrients in colorectal cancer in women, there appears to emerge a puzzling dichotomy between the results of the only two prospective cohort studies in women, the Nurses' Health Study and the Iowa Women's Health Study. Although both cohort studies used the same dietary assessment questionnaire, the results obtained for a number of dietary factors were not similar. For dietary fat and red meat, there was a direct association with colon cancer risk in the Nurses' Study and a null association in the Iowa Study. For dairy foods, calcium, and vitamin D intakes, there was no association in the Nurses' Study and a nonsignificant decrease after multivariate adjustment in the Iowa Study. However, in two smaller studies, an analysis of Utah women showed a halving of risk, and a similar decrease was seen in an Australian study as well. For antioxidant vitamins, the Iowa Study found total vitamin E intake to be inversely associated with risk for colorectal cancer, which seemed to decrease with age, whereas there was no association seen in the Nurses' Health Study.

The influence of increased fruit and vegetable consumption on colorectal cancer risk in women was analyzed in the Iowa Women's Health Study, and a decrease in risk was found. In the Nurses' Health Study, only vegetable and fruit fiber intakes were analyzed, and only fiber from fruit was associated with any appreciable reduction in risk; the overall trend did not attain statistical significance.

In summary, we appear to have a dilemma. The same diet questionnaire was administered to two different groups of women, and contrasting results have emerged from almost every dietary variable studied. This certainly leaves the general public totally confused as to what recommendations can be followed for a healthy, cancer-preventive diet. There are differences, however, between the two cohorts: the Nurses' Health Study was limited to women who were 30–55 years old and were registered nurses living in 11 large U.S. states,[40] whereas the Iowa Women's Health Study was limited to 55- to 69-year-old women living in a single state but in any occupational status or occupation.[41] Null associations in some studies could be due to dietary homogeneity within populations, either as a result of similarity in educational/occupational level (as in the Nurses' Study) or similarity due to narrow geographic isolation (as in the Iowa Study). Only speculative explanations can be attempted here, with so few women's studies available for a larger comparison beyond the two cohort studies. However, in the future, we should have a wealth of data on women's dietary habits, with both the Women's Health Initiative and the Women's Health Study (see Chapter 8) utilizing dietary information and interventions on a total of 140,000 women from all across the United States, representing all occupations. Future research on colorectal cancer in both gender studies should analyze separately by gender, so that there will be more of a database specific to colorectal cancer in women. Perhaps then we can reliably determine what the real dietary factors may be and how they may impact women differently than men.

REFERENCES

1. Parker, S.L., Tong, T., Bolden, S., and Wingo, P.A., Cancer statistics 1997, *CA Cancer J. Clin.*, 47, 5, 1997.
2. Cooper, H.S. and Slemmer, J.R., Surgical pathology of carcinoma of the colon and rectum, *Semin. Oncol.*, 18, 367, 1991.
3. Astler, V.B. and Coller, F.A., The prognostic significance of direct extension of carcinoma of the colon and rectum, *Ann. Surg.*, 139, 846, 1954.
4. Kyriakos, M., The President's cancer, the Dukes classification, and confusion, *Arch. Pathol. Lab. Med.*, 109, 1063, 1985.
5. Cotran, R.S., Kumar, V., and Robbins, S.L., *Robbins Pathologic Basis of Disease*, 5th ed., W.B. Saunders, Philadelphia, 1994, 817.
6. Schottenfeld, D. and Winawer, S.J., Cancers of the large intestine, in *Cancer Epidemiology and Prevention*, Schottenfeld, D. and Fraumeni, J.F., Jr., Eds., Oxford University Press, New York, 1996, chap. 39.
7. Herrera, L., Kakati, S., Gibas, L., Pietrzak, E., and Sandberg, A.A., Gardner's syndrome in a man with an intestinal deletion of 5q, *Am. J. Med. Genet.*, 25, 473, 1986.
8. Groden, J., Thiliveris, A., and Samowitz, W., Identification and characterization of the familial adenomatous polyposis coli gene, *Cell*, 66, 589, 1991.
9. Murday, V. and Slack, J., Inherited disorders associated with colorectal cancer, *Cancer Surv.*, 8, 139, 1989.
10. Konishi, M., Kikuchi-Yanoshita, R., Tanaka, K., Muraoka, M., Onda, A., Okumura, Y., Kishi, N., Iwama, T., Mori, T., Koike, M., Ushio, K., Chiba, M., Nomizu, S., Konishi, F., Utsunomiya, J., and Miyaki, M., Molecular nature of colon tumors in hereditary non-polyposis colon cancer, familial polyposis, and sporadic colon cancer, *Gastroenterology*, 111, 307, 1996.
11. Vogelstein, B., Fearon, E.R., Hamilton, S.R., Kern, S.E., Preisinger, A.C., Leppert, M., Nakamura, Y., White, R., Smits, A.M.M., and Bos, J.L., Genetic alterations during colorectal-tumor development, *New Engl. J. Med.*, 319, 525, 1988.
12. Fearon, E.R. and Vogelstein, B., A genetic model for colorectal tumorigenesis, *Cell*, 61, 759, 1990.
13. Peltomaki, P., Aaltonen, L.A., Sistonen, P., Pylkkanen, L., Mecklin, J.-P., Jarvinen, H., Green, J.S., Jass, J.R., Weber, J.L., Leach, F.S., Peterson, G.M., Hamilton, S.R., de la Chappelle, A., and Vogelstein, B., Genetic mapping of a locus predisposing to human colorectal cancer, *Science*, 260, 810, 1993.
14. Aaltonen, L., Peltomaki, P., Leach, F.S., Sistonen, P., Pylkkanen, L., Mecklin, J.-P., Jarvinen, H., Powell, S.M., Jen, J., Hamilton, S.R., Peterson, G.M., Kinzler, K.W., Vogelstein, B., and de la Chappelle, A., Clues to the pathogenesis of familial colorectal cancer, *Science*, 260, 812, 1993.
15. Thibodeau, S.N., Bren, G., and Schaid, D., Microsatellite instability in cancer of the proximal colon, *Science*, 260, 816, 1993.

16. Loeb, L.A., Microsatellite instability: marker of a mutator phenotype in cancer, *Cancer Res.*, 54, 5059, 1994.

17. Lewis, C.M., Neuhausen, S.L., Daley, D., Black, F.J., Swenson, J., Burt, R.W., Cannon-Albright, L.A., and Skolnick, M.H., Genetic heterogeneity and unmapped genes for colorectal cancer, *Cancer Res.*, 56, 1382, 1996.

18. DiVinci, A., Infusini, E., Reveri, C., Risio, M., Rossini, F.P., and Giaretti, W., Deletions at chromosome 1p by fluorescence *in situ* hybridization are an early event in human colorectal tumorigenesis, *Gastroenterology*, 111, 102, 1996.

19. DeJong, U.W., Day, N.E., Muir, C.S., Barclay, T.H., Bras, G., Foster, F.H., Jussawalla, D.J., Ringertz, N., and Shanmugaratnam, T., The distribution of cancer within the large bowel, *Int. J. Cancer*, 10, 463, 1972.

20. McMichael, A.J. and Potter, J.D., Reproduction, endogenous and exogenous sex hormones, and colon cancer: a review and hypothesis, *J. Natl. Cancer Inst.*, 65, 1201, 1980.

21. Fraumeni, J.F., Jr., Lloyd, J.W., Smith, E.M., and Wagoner, J.K., Cancer mortality among nuns: role of marital status in etiology of neoplastic disease in women, *J. Natl. Cancer Inst.*, 42, 455, 1969.

22. Weiss, N.S., Daling, J.R., and Chow, W.H., Incidence of cancer of the large bowel in women in relation to reproductive and hormonal factors, *J. Natl. Cancer Inst.*, 67, 57, 1981.

23. Potter, J.D. and McMichael, A.J., Large-bowel cancer in relation to reproductive and hormonal factors: a case-control study, *J. Natl. Cancer Inst.*, 71, 703, 1983.

24. Howe, G.R., Craib, K.J., and Miller, A.B., Age at first pregnancy and risk of colorectal cancer: a case-control study, *J. Natl. Cancer Inst.*, 74, 1155, 1985.

25. Wu, A.H., Paganini-Hill, A., Ross, R.K., and Henderson, B.E., Alcohol, physical activity, and other risk factors for colorectal cancer: a prospective study, *Br. J. Cancer*, 55, 687, 1987.

26. Martinez, M.E., Grodstein, F., Giovanucci, E., Colditz, G.A., Speizer, F.E., Hennekens, C., Rosner, B., Willett, W.C., and Stampfer, M.J., A prospective study of reproductive factors, oral contraceptive use, and risk of colorectal cancer, *Cancer Epidemiol. Biomarkers Prev.*, 6, 1, 1997.

27. Potter, J.D., Hormones and colon cancer: editorial, *J. Natl. Cancer Inst.*, 87, 1039, 1995.

28. Wu-Williams, A.H., Lee, M., Whittemore, A.S., Gallagher, R.P., Deng-ao, J., Shu, Z., Lun, Z., Xianghui, W., Kun, C., Jung, D., The, C.-Z., Chengde, L., Yao, X.J., Paffenbarger, R.S., Jr., and Henderson, B.E., Reproductive factors and colorectal cancer risk among Chinese females, *Cancer Res.*, 51, 2307, 1991.

29. Risch, H.A. and Howe, G.R., Menopausal hormone use and colorectal cancer in Saskatchewan: a record linkage cohort study, *Cancer Epidemiol. Biomarkers Prev.*, 4, 21, 1995.

30. Calle, E.E., Miracle-McMahill, H.L., Thun, M.J., and Heath, C.W., Jr., Estrogen replacement therapy and risk of fatal colon cancer in a prospective cohort of postmenopausal women, *J. Natl. Cancer Inst.*, 87, 517, 1995.

31. Newcomb, P.A. and Storer, B.E., Postmenopausal hormone use and risk of large-bowel cancer, *J. Natl. Cancer Inst.*, 87, 1067, 1995.

32. Potter, J.D., Bostick, R.M., Grandits, G.A., Fosdick, L., Elmer, P., Wood, J., Grambsch, P., and Louis, T.A., Hormone replacement therapy is associated with lower risk of adenomatous polyps of the large bowel: the Minnesota Cancer

Prevention Research Unit case-control study, *Cancer Epidemiol. Biomarkers Prev.*, 5, 779, 1996.

33. Giovanucci, E., Colditz, G.A., Stampfer, M.J., Hunter, D., Rosner, B.A., Willett, W.C., and Speizer, F.E., A prospective study of cigarette smoking and risk of colorectal adenoma and colorectal cancer in U.S. women, *J. Natl. Cancer Inst.*, 86, 192, 1994.

34. Chute, C.G., Willett, W.C., Colditz, G.A., Stampfer, M.J., Baron, J.A., Rosner, B., and Speizer, F.E., A prospective study of body mass, height, and smoking on the risk of colorectal cancer in women, *Cancer Causes Control*, 2, 117, 1991.

35. Giovannucci, E. and Martinez, M.E., Tobacco, colorectal cancer and adenomas: a review of the evidence, *J. Natl. Cancer Inst.*, 88, 1717, 1996.

36. Reeves, M.J., Newcomb, P.A., Trentham-Dietz, A., Storer, B.E., and Remington, P.L., Nonsteroidal anti-inflammatory drug use and protection against colorectal cancer in women, *Cancer Epidemiol. Biomarkers Prev.*, 5, 955, 1996.

37. Slattery, M.L., Potter, J.D., Caan, B., Edwards, S., Coates, A., Ma, K.-N., and Berry, T.D., Energy balance and colon cancer—beyond physical activity, *Cancer Res.*, 57, 75, 1997.

38. Shoff, S.M., Newcomb, P.A., and Longnecker, M.P., Frequency of eating and risk of colorectal cancer in women, *Nutr. Cancer*, 27, 22, 1997.

39. Potter, J.D., Slattery, M.L., Bostick, R.M., and Gapstur, S.M., Colon cancer: a review of the epidemiology, *Epidemiol. Rev.*, 15, 199, 1993.

40. Willett, W.C., Stampfer, M.J., Colditz, G.A., Rosner, B.A., and Speizer, F.E., Relation of meat, fat, and fiber intake to the risk of colon cancer in a prospective study among women, *New Engl. J. Med.*, 323, 1664, 1990.

41. Bostick, R.M., Potter, J.D., Steinmetz, K.A., Kushi, L.H., Sellars, T.A., McKenzie, D.R., Gapstur, S.M., and Folsom, A.R., Sugar, meat, and fat intake and non-dietary risk factors for colon cancer incidence in Iowa women (United States), *Cancer Causes Control*, 5, 38, 1994.

42. Willett, W.C. and Stampfer, M.J., Total energy intake: implications for the epidemiologic analyses, *Am. J. Epidemiol.*, 124, 17, 1986.

43. Gerhardsson de Verdier, M., Hagman, U., Peters, R.K., Steineck, G., and Overvik, E., Meat, cooking methods and colorectal cancer: a case-referent study in Stockholm, *Int. J. Cancer*, 49, 520, 1991.

44. Bostick, R.M., Diet and nutrition in the etiology and primary prevention of colon cancer, in *Prevention: The Comprehensive Guide for Health Professionals*, Bendich, A. and Decklebaum, R.J., Eds., Humana Press, Totawa, NJ, 1997, chap. 4.

45. Bostick, R.M., Potter, J.D., Sellers, T.A., McKenzie, D.R., Kushi, L.H., and Folsom, A.R., Relation of calcium, vitamin D, and dairy food intake to incidence of colon cancer among older women: the Iowa Women's Health Study, *Am. J. Epidemiol.*, 137, 1302, 1993.

46. Slattery, M.L., Sorenson, A.W., and Ford, M.H., Dietary calcium as a mitigating factor in colon cancer, *Am. J. Epidemiol.*, 128, 504, 1988.

47. Kune, S., Kune, G.M., and Watson, F., Case-control study of dietary etiologic factors: the Melbourne Colorectal Cancer Study, *Nutr. Cancer*, 9, 21, 1987.

48. Kampman, E., Giovannucci, E., van't Veer, P., Rimm, E., Stampfer, M.J., Colditz, G.A., Kok, F.J., and Willett, W.C., Calcium, vitamin D, dairy foods, and the

occurrence of colorectal adenomas among men and women in two prospective studies, *Am. J. Epidemiol.*, 139, 16, 1994.

49. Bostick, R.M., Potter, J.D., McKenzie, D.R., Sellers, T.A., Kushi, L.H., Steinmetz, K.A., and Folsom, A.R., Reduced risk of colon cancer with high intake of vitamin E: the Iowa Women's Health Study, *Cancer Res.*, 53, 4230, 1993.

50. Willett, W.C., Sampson, L., Browne, M.L., Stampfer, M.J., Rosner, B., Hennekens, C.H., and Speizer, F.E., The use of a self-administered questionnaire to assess diet 4 years in the past, *Am. J. Epidemiol.*, 127, 188, 1988.

51. Greenberg, E.R., Baron, J.A., Tosteson, T.D., Freeman, D.H., Beck, G.J., Bond, J.H., Colacchio, T.A., Coller, J.A., Frankl, H.D., Haile, R.W., Mandel, J.S., Nierenberg, D.W., Rothstein, R., Snover, D.C., Stevens, M.M., Summers, R.W., and van Stolk, R.U., A clinical trial of antioxidant vitamins to prevent colorectal adenoma, *New Engl. J. Med.*, 331, 141, 1994.

52. Longnecker, M.P., Martin-Moreno, J., Knekt, P., Nomura, A.M.Y., Schober, S.E., Stahellin, H.B., Wald, N.J., Gey, K.F., and Willett, W.C., Serum alpha-tocopherol concentrations in relation to subsequent colorectal cancer: pooled data from five cohorts, *J. Natl. Cancer Inst.*, 84, 430, 1992.

53. Clark, L.C., Combs, G.F., Turnbull, B.W., Slate, E.H., Chalker, D.K., Chow, D., Davis, L.S., Glover, R.A., Graham, G.F., Gross, E.G., Krongrad, A., Lesher, J.L., Park, H.K., Sanders, B.B., Smith, C.L., and Taylor, J.R., Effects of selenium supplementation for cancer prevention in patients with carcinoma of the skin: a randomized controlled trial, *J. Am. Med. Assoc.*, 276, 1957, 1996.

54. Clark, L.C., Hixson, L.J., Combs, G.F., Jr., Reid, M.E., Turnbull, B.W., and Sampliner, R.E., Plasma selenium concentration predicts the prevalence of colorectal adenomatous polyps, *Cancer Epidemiol. Biomarkers Prev.*, 2, 41, 1993.

55. Potter, J.D. and McMichael, A.J., Diet and cancer of the colon and rectum: a case-control study, *J. Natl. Cancer Inst.*, 76, 557, 1986.

56. Lyon, J.L., Mahoney, A.W., West, D.W. Gardner, J.W., Smith, K.R., Sorenson, A.W., and Stanish, W., Energy intake: its relationship to colon cancer risk, *J. Natl. Cancer Inst.*, 78, 853, 1987.

57. West, D.W., Slattery, M.L., Robison, L.M., Schuman, K.L., Ford, M.H., Mahoney, A.W., Lyon, J.D., and Sorenson, A.W., Dietary intake and colon cancer: sex and anatomic site-specific associations, *Am. J. Epidemiol.*, 130, 883, 1989.

58. Paganini-Hill, A., Chao, A., Ross, R.K., and Henderson, B.E., Vitamin A, beta-carotene and the risk of cancer: a prospective study, *J. Natl. Cancer Inst.*, 79, 443, 1987.

59. Heilbrun, L.K., Nomura, A., Hankin, J.H., and Stemmermann, G.N., Diet and colorectal cancer with special reference to fiber intake, *Int. J. Cancer*, 44, 1, 1989.

60. Enger, S.M., Longnecker, M.P., Chen, M.-J., Harper, J.M., Lee, E.R., Frankl, H.D., and Haile, R.W., Dietary intake of carotenoids and vitamins A, C, and E, and prevalence of colorectal adenomas, *Cancer Epidemiol. Biomarkers Prev.*, 5, 147, 1996.

61. Steinmetz, K.A. and Potter, J.D., Vegetables, fruit, and cancer. I. Epidemiology, *Cancer Causes Control*, 2, 325, 1991.

62. Steinmetz, K.A. and Potter, J.D., Vegetables, fruit, and cancer. II. Mechanisms, *Cancer Causes Control*, 2, 427, 1991.

63. Trock, B., Lanza, E., and Greenwald, P., Dietary fiber, vegetables, and colon cancer: critical review and meta-analyses of the epidemiologic evidence, *J. Natl. Cancer Inst.*, 82, 650, 1990.

64. Slattery, M.L., Sorenson, A.W., Mahoney, A.W., French, T.K., Kritchevsky, D., and Street, J.C., Diet and colon cancer: assessment of risk by fiber type and food source, *J. Natl. Cancer Inst.*, 80, 1474, 1988 (published erratum appears in *J. Natl. Cancer Inst.*, 81, 1042, 1989).

65. Graham, S., Marshall, J., Haughey, B., Mittelman, A., Swanson, M., Zielzeny, M., Byers, T., Wilkinson, G., and West, D., Dietary epidemiology of cancer of the colon in western New York, *Am. J. Epidemiol.*, 128, 490, 1988.

66. Reddy, B.S., Simi, B., and Engle, A., Biochemical epidemiology of colon cancer: effect of types of dietary fiber on colonic diacylglycerols in women, *Gastroenterology*, 106, 883, 1994.

67. Sandler, R.S., Lyles, C.M., Peipins, L.A., McAuliffe, C.A., Woosley, J.T., and Kupper, L.L., Diet and risk of colorectal adenomas: macronutrients, cholesterol, and fiber, *J. Natl. Cancer Inst.*, 85, 884, 1993.

68. Steinmetz, K.A., Kushi, L.H., Bostick, R.M., Folsom, A.R., and Potter, J.D., Vegetables, fruit, and colon cancer in the Iowa Women's Health Study, *Am. J. Epidemiol.*, 139, 1, 1994.

69. Frentzel-Beyme, R. and Chang-Claude, J., Vegetarian diets and colon cancer: the German experience, *Am. J. Clin. Nutr.*, 59, 1143S, 1994.

70. La Vecchia, C., Negri, E., Decarli, A., D'Avanza, B., Gallotti, L., Gentile, A., and Franceschi, S., A case-control study of diet and colorectal cancer in northern Italy, *Int. J. Cancer*, 41, 492, 1988.

71. Bristol, J.B., Emmett, P.M., Heaton, K.W., and Williamson, R.C.N., Sugar, fat, and the risk of colorectal cancer, *Br. Med. J.*, 291, 1467, 1985.

72. Marquart-Moulin, G., Riboli, E., Comee, J., Kaaks, R., and Berthezene, P., Colorectal polyps and diet: a case-control study in Marseilles, *Int. J. Cancer*, 40, 179, 1987.

73. Miller, A.B., Howe, G.R., Jain, M., Craib, K.J.P., and Harrison, L., Food items and food groups as risk factors in a case-control study of diet and colorectal cancer, *Int. J. Cancer*, 32, 155, 1983.

74. Giovannucci, E., Stampfer, M.J., Colditz, G.A., Rimm, E.B., Trichopoulos, D., Rosner, B.A., Speizer, F.E., and Willett, W.C., Folate, methionine, and alcohol intake and risk of colorectal adenomas, *J. Natl. Cancer Inst.*, 85, 875, 1993.

CHAPTER 7

NUTRITION AND LUNG CANCER IN WOMEN

CONTENTS

I. GENERAL PATHOLOGY AND STATISTICS

Lung cancer accounts for about 13% of all newly diagnosed cancers in women and 25% of all cancer-related deaths.[1] It is the fastest rising cause of cancer deaths in women, and the death rate has not yet peaked, as it has for men.[1]

According to the classification of bronchogenic carcinoma by the World Health Organization, there are four main subcategories of these tumors: squamous cell carcinoma (25–40%), adenocarcinoma (25–40%), small cell carcinoma (20–25%), and large cell carcinoma (10–15%).[2] There may be combinations of different cell types even in the same tumors.[3] It is expected that lung cancer will become the most common cause of cancer death in both men and women. It surpassed breast cancer as the leading cancer killer of women in 1987. It is a disease usually seen in the sixth decade of life, and only 2% of cases occur under the age of 40.

Squamous cell carcinoma demonstrates histologically keratin pearls with intercellular bridges (desmosomes) and ultrastructurally tonofilaments and diffuse keratin. Squamous cell carcinoma can arise anywhere in the bronchi, often near the hilum. Large squamous cell carcinomas tend to cavitate. Hemorrhage into the cavity and/or eroded bronchus can be the terminal event. Squamous metaplasia and dysplasia are often found in the bronchi surrounding a squamous carcinoma.

Adenocarcinoma usually demonstrates gland formation, papillae, mucin production histologically, and microvilli and secretory granules ultrastructurally. Adenocarcinoma is more common in women and can be seen in nonsmokers. It is often at the periphery of the lung. A primary lung adenocarcinoma may look identical to a metastasis from another organ. About 10% of adenocarcinomas are of the bronchioloalveolar subtype, considered to include cancers of the bronchial goblet cells, type II pneumocytes, and Clara cells. These malignant cells grow along the alveolar septal framework and secrete mucus into the alveoli.

Large-cell undifferentiated carcinoma demonstrates large cells with abundant cytoplasm, large vesicular nuclei histologically, and no distinct features ultrastructurally. Small cell undifferentiated carcinoma demonstrates histologically "small blue cells" with little cytoplasm and nuclear molding with "neurosecretory" granules usually seen ultrastructurally. Small-cell undifferentiated carcinomas arise anywhere in the lung, but most often occur near the hilum and, hence, can quickly spread along bronchi. Small-cell undifferentiated carcinoma can secrete many different substances, such as adrenocorticotrophic hormone and antidiuretic hormone.[4]

The new International Staging System for lung cancer is as follows:[5,6]

T1	Tumor <3 cm without pleural or mainstream bronchus involvement
T2	Tumor >3 cm or involvement of mainstream bronchus >2 cm from carina, visceral, pleural, or lobular atelectasis
T3	Tumor with involvement of chest wall (including superior sulcus tumors, diaphragm, mediastinal pleura, pericardium, mainstream bronchus <2 cm from carina, or entire lung atelectasis
T4	Tumor with invasion of mediastinum, heart, great vessels, trachea, esophagus, vertebral body, or carina or with malignant pleural effusion
N0	No demonstrable metastasis to regional lymph nodes
N1	Ipsilateral hilar or peribronchial nodal involvement
N2	Metastasis to ipsilateral mediastinal or subcarinal lymph nodes
N3	Metastasis to contralateral mediastinal or hilar lymph nodes, ipsilateral or contralateral scalene, or supraclavicular lymph nodes
M0	No (known) distant metastasis
M1	Distant metastasis present

Stage Grouping			
Stage I	T1–2	N0	M0
Stage II	T1–2	N1	M0
Stage IIIa	T1–3	N2	M0
	T3	N0–2	M0
Stage IIIb	Any	TN3	M0
	T4	Any N	M0
Stage IV	Any T	Any N	M1

From Cotran, R.S., Kumar, V., and Robbins, S.L., *Robbins Pathologic Basis of Disease*, 5th ed., W.B. Saunders, Philadelphia, 1994, 724. With permission.

The overall 5-year survival rate is on the order of 9%. Not more than 20–30% of lung cancer patients have lesions sufficiently localized to permit even an attempt at resection. The adenocarcinoma and squamous cell patterns tend to remain localized longer and have a slightly better prognosis than do the undifferentiated cancers, which usually are advanced lesions by the time they are discovered. The overall 5-year survival rate of males is approximately 10% for squamous cell carcinoma and adenocarcinoma, but only 3% for undifferentiated lesions. The survival time for patients with small cell cancer is about 1 year. The outlook is poor for most patients with bronchogenic carcinoma.[6]

II. POPULATION GENETICS AND MARKERS FOR RISK

Squamous cell carcinoma and small cell lung carcinoma (SCLC) are the histological types of lung cancer most associated with cigarette smoking, and they tend to develop in the proximal airways. Adenocarcinomas and bronchioalveolar carcinomas tend to develop more distally in the terminal bronchioles or alveoli.[7] A clinical distinction is often drawn between SCLC and non-SCLC, since SCLCs typically are chemoresponsive and highly metastatic early in their course and non-SCLCs usually are less responsive and more of a local problem.[7] A number of dominant and recessive oncogenes have been examined for their role in the etiology of lung cancer. Somatic mutations have been found in *ras* genes in human lung cancer. Carbone and Minna[7] have summarized the results from a number of large studies of *ras* in lung cancer and have found that they occur in 31% of adenocarcinomas and 21% of large cell cancers, but are found in only 5% of squamous cell carcinomas and are not found in SCLC.[7] Most *ras* mutations are found in adenocarcinomas and almost predominantly at Ki-*ras* codon 12. Carbone and Minna[7] have summarized these data and have found that 30 of 46 tumors examined had codon 12 mutations, and very few were found in other codons. The presence of a *ras* mutation has also been reported to be an unfavorable prognostic factor in early-stage adenocarcinomas.[8]

The involvement of the *myc* genes in human lung cancer has not been found to be associated with gene mutations, but with amplification and/or overexpression of the gene. The studies of this gene in lung cancer have reported frequencies of amplification in SCLC which range from 10 to 100%.[7] This amplification is also associated with poorer clinical outcome as well.[9] Overexpression seems to be more common than amplification and has been seen in 16 of 18 tumors in one study.[10] Amplification of the *myc* gene is rare in non-SCLC, and only 2 of 47 tumor samples were positive in one study.[11] Other dominant oncogenes that have been examined in lung cancer would include Her-2/*neu*, gastrin-releasing peptide receptor, and c-*myb*,[7] although none of these appears to play a prominent role.

Recessive oncogenes or tumor suppressor genes also appear to play a role in the etiology of lung cancer. Frequent abnormalities in the *Rb* gene have been reported in SCLC and with much less frequency in non-SCLC.[12] Non-SCLC appears to have abnormal Rb protein in about 20% of cases.[7] Abnormalities in the *p53* tumor suppressor gene appear to be frequent events in lung cancer.[13] Recent studies have reported a 42% frequency of *p53* mutations, with those predominantly occurring in squamous cell carcinoma and in younger patients.[14] However, the picture in SCLC is that 100% of tumors may have abnormal *p53*.[7] The most common codon for mutation in *p53* is 273 for all tumor types combined, and for non-SCLC tumors, G-to-T transversions are the most common base change in the *p53* gene.[7]

There also appears to be a link between loss of a specific site on chromosome 3p in over 90% of informative cases of SCLC.[15] This has proved to be an elusive cancer susceptibility gene in that attempts to identify this putative recessive oncogene on chromosome 3p have met with little success to date.[15] Although researchers have been unable to define a minimum consensus deletion by RFLP analyses in lung cancer, it is known that there is a fragile site at 3p14 which is associated with increased breakage and sister chromatid exchange in the peripheral blood and bone marrow of young cigarette smokers.[16]

Although there is a strong association of lung cancer with the environmental risk factors of tobacco abuse and radon and asbestos exposure, there may also be an inherited predisposition to lung cancer risk. A recent study of family history and lung cancer risk demonstrated a 2.4-fold overall excess risk to relatives of lung cancer patients, even after adjusting for all known environmental factors.[17] However, when specific oncogenes are examined in non-tumor DNA from lung cancer patients, there does not appear to be strong support for the hypothesis of germline mutations increasing risk in families. However, since tobacco carcinogenesis is a complex interaction between a cancer-causing agent and the human host, metabolism of these carcinogens is a factor in predisposition to the resulting cancer. A major pathway of carcinogen metabolic activation involving the CYP2D6 enzyme of the P450 group appears to have a specific association with lung cancer susceptibility.[7] CYP2D6 is an enzyme called debrisoquine hydroxylase. In one study, individuals who are of the extensive metabolizer phenotype for debrisoquine showed a tenfold increased risk for lung cancer.[18] Additionally, abnormal gene regulation of the

CYP1A1 enzyme has been reported in lung cancer.[19] Carcinogen detoxification enzyme capabilities are also linked to lung cancer risk, especially the Phase II enzyme glutathione-S-transferase M1 (GSTM1).[20] A lack of the GSTM1 or the null phenotype is a risk factor for squamous cell carcinoma of the lung.[20] Thus, we see that although there does not appear to be a strong direct oncogenetic component linked to risk for lung cancer, the inherent ability of the individual to metabolize the carcinogens in tobacco smoke is an important determinant of risk.

III. GENERAL EPIDEMIOLOGY OF LUNG CANCER IN WOMEN

A. Cigarette Smoking

In the 1920s and 1930s, an alarming increase in lung cancer incidence, along with clinical observations, raised the suspicion that smoking might be a causal factor. Case-control studies in the United States and Great Britain appeared in the early 1950s supporting this hypothesis.[21] In 1964 the Surgeon General of the United States issued a report on smoking and essentially declared that cigarette smoking was the major cause of lung cancer in American men.[21] These first reports were concerned only with male smokers, but as female smoking habits have approached the same levels as men, the lung cancer rates for women have risen accordingly.

Female lung cancer mortality rates have increased 500% since 1950, and lung cancer became the leading cause of cancer death in U.S. women in 1987, as it has been for men since the 1950s.[22] Today, as already stated, it accounts for 25% of female cancer deaths, compared with only 3% in 1950. Lung cancer survival rates are slightly more favorable in female than male patients, but are generally poor and have improved only slightly in the past few decades.[22] In women as in men, lung cancer has reached epidemic proportions following the widespread acceptance of cigarette smoking, with a lag time of 20–30 years between adoption of the practice and the emergence of the cancer. Currently, at least 80% of female and 90% of male lung cancer deaths in the United States are attributable to smoking.[22] A number of studies in recent years have calculated relative risks for smoking and the different histologic types of cancer (for review, see Blot and Fraumeni[21]), and it has been shown that smoking increases the risk of all histologic types, but the effect appears to be greater for small cell cancers, followed by squamous cell and then adenocarcinomas.[22]

B. Environmental Tobacco Smoke and Other Factors

Environmental tobacco smoke (ETS) has been designated as a group A carcinogen by the U.S. Environmental Protection Agency, thus concluding that

ETS causes lung cancer in nonsmokers. There are over 30 epidemiologic studies worldwide which have compared the risk of lung cancer in nonsmoking women married to men who smoke to the risks for those women who are married to men who do not smoke. Although many of these studies showed rather modest relative risks or no association, the EPA has estimated that 3.9% of the female lung cancer deaths in the United States are attributable to ETS.[23]

Other environmental factors as well play a role in the disease, such as exposure to asbestos, ionizing radiation, arsenic, and polycyclic aromatic hydrocarbons.[22] Those that have been particularly studied in women include residential radon exposure and indoor air pollution from coal-burning stoves, especially in China. However, most studies of radon exposure only find increased odds ratios among smokers.[22]

Throughout the world, the incidence of lung cancer among men exceeds, usually by twofold or more, that among women, among whom annual age-adjusted rates are generally below 40 per 100,000.[21] This sex difference has usually been attributed to the lower smoking prevalence by females compared with males, although this gender difference is apparently shrinking. The male/female ratio for lung cancer is lowest in parts of China, where there are the world's highest rates of lung cancer in women, especially adenocarcinoma.[24, 25] In the United States, cancer incidence trends in women show a 122.4% change in lung and bronchus cancer incidence from 1973 to 1993.[26] Overall cancer incidence has increased 13.7% in that time frame, and the rise in lung cancer incidence accounts for most of that rise. When lung cancer incidence is excluded, the overall rise in cancer incidence in U.S. women is only 6.4%.[26] Lung cancer incidence is gradually leveling off in U.S. men, but is continuing to rise in women. In the United States, the rise in lung cancer incidence is largely attributed to smoking patterns in women.

C. Increased Female Susceptibility to Lung Carcinogens

The significant increase in lung cancer deaths in women since 1950 may, however, be due to more than increased smoking.[27] Although there has been a 500% increase in female lung cancer mortality since 1950,[28] presumably due to changed smoking patterns, a very recent study by Zang and Wynder[29] suggests that women may be more susceptible to DNA damage from carcinogen exposure than are men. Recent epidemiological studies have reported that, dose for dose, women may be more susceptible to tobacco carcinogens than are men.[30–33] The most recent investigation of gender differences in lung cancer risk examined data from 1889 cases with lung cancer of all types, except mesothelioma, and 2070 controls with diseases unrelated to smoking.[29] Their results indicated that women were more likely to be never-smokers than men, especially for those with squamous/epidermoid-type cancers. Men also started smoking earlier, reported greater inhalation, and smoked more cigarettes per day than did women.[29] However, the dose–response odds ratios over cumulative exposure to cigarette smoking were significantly higher (1.2- to 1.7-fold higher) in women than in men for the three major histological types of lung cancer. These results held even after adjustment for weight, height, and body mass index. The authors concluded that these data confirm their earlier findings that odds ratios for lung cancer types are consistently higher for women than for men at every level of cigarette exposure, and that these results are consistent with the implication that women are more susceptible to tobacco carcinogens than are men.[29] Concurrence with these findings has also been recently reported by Cohn et al.[34] from a small cohort study which also showed that cigarette smoking is a stronger predictor of lung cancer among women than among men.

There are a number of factors which could account for gender differences in susceptibility to lung cancer from cigarette smoking exposure. These might include gender differences in nicotine metabolism, male–female differences in cytochrome P450 enzymes, and the effect of estrogenic hormones on lung tumor development.[29] Several clinical studies have shown that the total clearance of nicotine, adjusted for body weight, is lower in women than in men.[35, 36] However, another study done in the United Kingdom[37] found no gender differences in nicotine exposure. There are a number of CYP450 forms that are involved in the bioactivation of the cigarette smoke carcinogens, and there have been some reports which indicate that there might be sex differences in how these compounds are metabolized, although most studies have been in experimental animals.[29] Finally, the influence of estrogen has been studied in women who are taking hormone replacement therapy, and it has been found that, in general, those with supplemental estrogen have an elevated relative risk for lung cancer.[29] It is also known that estrogen affects CYP450 metabolism in experimental animals.[29, 38] In summary, it appears that there are several plausible mechanisms whereby women might be more susceptible to carcinogenesis by tobacco smoke exposure than are men.

IV. DIETARY FACTORS AND LUNG CANCER IN WOMEN

A. Cholesterol and/or Dietary Fat

A number of recent case-control epidemiologic investigations have suggested that a high consumption of cholesterol and/or dietary fat may be associated with an elevated risk for lung cancer (Table 7.1).[39–43] In cohort studies, however, only one demonstrated a positive association,[44] but two others showed no association.[45, 46] Most of these dietary studies did not include women, and those that did had only small numbers of female cases. The most comprehensive study of dietary cholesterol and fat intake in women was an analysis of

Jle 7.1   Studies of Nutrition and Lung Cancer in Women Only

Nutrient	Type of Study	Association with Risk	Reference
Cholesterol, saturated fat intake	Case-control	Direct	43
Cholesterol, fat	IWHS[a]	No association	47
Fruits and vegetables	IWHS	Decreased by half, better for ex-smokers	64
	Case-control	Decreased risk in nonsmokers	66
	Case-control	Decreased risk in passive smoking, relative risk = 0.27	57
Vegetables intake	Case-control	Decreased risk in light and never-smokers	54
	Case-control	Decreased risk in never-smokers	52, 57
All vegetables	Case-control	Decreased risk of death	67
Fresh fruit, fresh fish	Case-control	Decreased risk in never-smokers	52
Carotenoid vegetables	Case-control	No association	72
Carotene, total vegetables	Case-control	Decreased risk, odds ratio = 0.3 and 0.2 respectively, never-smokers	73
Retinol intake	Case-control	No association	73
Vitamin C intake	Case-control	Decreased, nonsignificant	73

[a] IWHS = Iowa Women's Health Study, a prospective cohort study.

dietary data from the Iowa Women's Health Study, which was conducted among 41,837 postmenopausal Iowa women.[47] The Iowa Women's Health Study is a prospective cohort study among Iowa women in which a mailed questionnaire was completed in 1986. This cohort was followed for cancer incidence through the SEER program, and after 6 years of follow-up, 272 incident cases of lung cancer were confirmed.[47] The histologic type of these cancers was 42.0% squamous or small cell carcinomas, 36.3% adenocarcinomas, and 21.7% were of unknown or other types, such as large cell carcinomas.[47] A total of 212 cases were included in the analyses. The exposures analyzed were dietary cholesterol and fat intake. With the exception of plant-derived fat, no significant association was observed between dietary cholesterol or fat intake and lung cancer risk in postmenopausal women. This was the only significant P for trend observed, and the relative risk for the highest quartile of intake among smokers was 0.7 for all cases and no significant trends by histological type. However, when the data were further adjusted for smoking status, there were no associations between lung cancer risk and cholesterol and total animal or plant fat intakes. The authors concluded that their data do not support an etiologic link between these nutrients and lung cancer in women.[47]

B. Fruits and Vegetables

The most consistent association in diet and lung cancer risk has been that for consumption of fresh vegetables and fruits and lowered risk. Twelve case-control studies have reported an inverse association of fruits and vegetables with lung cancer risk, and fewer cohort studies have done so.[39, 48–61] However, most of these studies have been in men. We know from our discussion above that the risks for lung cancer are different for men and women,[29] that the attributable risk for smoking is lower for women, that this cancer is diagnosed at a younger age in women, and that survival is generally better than for men.[62, 63] For these reasons, it is important to analyze the effects of vegetable and fruit intake in a population of only women. Steinmetz et al.[64] have examined the impact of fruit and vegetable intake in the Iowa Women's Health Study, where 179 cases of lung cancer had developed by the time of the study. In this prospective study of postmenopausal women, the risk of lung cancer was decreased by half in the highest quartile of consumption of all vegetables and fruit, all vegetables, and green leafy vegetables, compared with the lowest quartile of intake.[64] Adjusted odds ratios were 0.49, 0.50, 0.75, and 0.45 for all vegetables and fruit, all vegetables, all fruit, and green leafy vegetables, respectively, after adjustment for age, energy intake, and pack-years of smoking.[64] In general, these associations were strongest for large cell carcinoma and stronger for ex-smokers than for current smokers.[64]

Several other studies that also separated effects according to gender reported results in partial agreement with the Steinmetz et al. study. Le Marchand et al.[54] reported on both males and females in their study of vegetable consumption and lung cancer risk in a case-control study in Hawaii. They found that vegetable consumption was more associated with reduced risk in light smokers and never-smokers in females, whereas the association was strongest in heavy and current smokers in males.[54] Koo[52] and Kalandidi et al.[57] have also reported separate results for females and have found protective effects of fruit and vegetable consumption in those who have never smoked.

1. Diet and Lung Cancer in Nonsmokers

A number of recent studies have examined the roles of diet and passive smoking in the risk for lung cancer among nonsmoking women. Matonoski et al.[65] examined the relationship between passive smoking and diet in 3896 nonsmoking women from the NHANES I data. They found no difference between exposed and nonexposed women in the levels of fatty acid intake or intake of other foods from the food frequency list in terms of general dietary habits. However, there were many nondietary differences between those women exposed to passive smoke and those not exposed. The exposed women tended to be older, less educated, urban dwelling, and have other risky health behaviors. Mayne et al.[66] examined diet and lung cancer risk in a group of nonsmoking women. These authors pointed out that 15% of lung cancer deaths cannot be attributed to cigarette smoking and that increased consumption of vegetables, raw fruits and vegetables, and dairy products decreased the risk of nonsmoking-associated lung cancer in this population of females.[66] Kalandidi al.[57] had earlier examined the role of passive smoking and diet in a Greek population of nonsmoking women in Athens. They reported that the relative risk for lung cancer for women married to smokers was 2.1 and increased with the duration of the exposure time and number of cigarettes smoked per day. As for the dietary data, they reported that a high consumption of fruits and vegetables decreased this passive smoking risk (relative risk with highest quartile of intake was 0.27). Neither vegetables nor any other specific food groups provided additional protective effects. These authors concluded that the apparent protective effect of vegetables seen in other studies was thus not due only to carotenoid vitamin A intake and was only partly explained in terms of vitamin C. Other studies of nonsmoking women relate more specifically to beta-carotene and will be discussed in the following section.

Koo[52] had examined in a retrospective case-control study in Hong Kong the dietary habits and lung cancer risk among Chinese females who never smoked tobacco. Lung cancer among females in Hong Kong is notable because it had the highest age-adjusted incidence rate in the world in 1982, and 64% of the cases were found not to be attributable to smoking.[52] Those in the lowest tertile of intake of fresh fruit or fresh fish had significantly elevated relative risks of 2.4 and 2.8, respectively. Interestingly, these protective effects were largely confined to those with adenocarcinoma or large cell tumors.[52]

Goodman et al.[67] studied the role of diet and lung cancer survival in men and women. They reported that their food group analysis showed a significant decrease in the risk of death from lung cancer with increasing consumption of all vegetables combined among women, but not among men. Similarly, the association of fruit intake with increased survival was seen among women, but not in men. Specific food items which showed a positive association with increased survival among women specifically were broccoli and tomatoes. The authors concluded that certain components of fruits and vegetables may prolong survival in female lung cancer patients.

C. The Beta-Carotene Story

A large number of epidemiologic investigations have been published on the risks of lung cancer associated with dietary beta-carotene intake, and these have been meticulously collected and presented by Blot and Fraumeni.[21] In general, most of these dietary intake studies have shown a protective effect in a number of different populations from all over the world. However, most of these studies have involved males, and there are few female-only analyses. Those studies that have been exclusively in females have been singled out specifically in this chapter. Also, a number of biochemical studies have demonstrated reduced levels of beta-carotene in stored sera from those persons who later developed lung cancer.[21] Carotenoid intake, as well as serum beta-carotene concentrations, seem to be lower in smokers, and some have reported that the protective effects of carotenoids may be greater among current and recent smokers.[21]

The sum total of the observational epidemiologic data on beta-carotene and lung cancer risk prompted two notable intervention trials. The Alpha-Tocopherol, Beta-Carotene Trial was a randomized intervention trial among 29,133 male smokers in Finland.[68] However, following up to 8 years of supplementation with 20 mg/day of beta-carotene, the study actually showed an 18% increase in lung cancers and an 8% increase in deaths in those on the beta-carotene. At the time this study was published, it was thought that these results might even be due to chance. However, another trial in the United States was conducted with an intervention of daily supplementation with 30 mg of beta-carotene plus 25,000 IU of retinol.[69] This was the Beta-Carotene and Retinol Efficacy Trial (CARET), which applied the intervention to both male and female heavy smokers and male asbestos workers. This trial had to be stopped 21 months early because 28% more of the participants taking the carotene/retinol intervention got lung cancer than did those on the placebo.[70] These findings raise the possibility that correlates of beta-carotene have been responsible for the protective effects seen in the prior epidemiologic studies.[21] However, in contrast, the Physicians' Health Study, in which 22,071 male physicians in the United States took aspirin or beta-carotene for over 12 years, showed a small 7% reduction in lung cancer. However, the population chosen for this particular intervention was at low risk for lung cancer.[71] These findings in such large trials underscore the need to further define the protective components in fruits and vegetables and also raise the question of whether beta-carotene consumption might only be a marker for a more healthy lifestyle. Also, since most of these interventions have taken place in male-only trials, there is a need to determine if the above-mentioned effects also apply to women smokers.

Wu-Williams et al.[72] performed a case-control study of lung cancer among females only in two cities in China with the highest lung cancer rates in that country. They found that cigarette smoking was the main causal factor and accounted for 35% of lung cancers in this population.[72] Air pollution from coal-burning stoves was also implicated, as was occupational exposure from working in a smelter. Interestingly, this study did not find a protective effect of carotene-rich vegetables in this population. In contrast, Candelora et al.[73] conducted a case-control study to examine the influence of dietary factors on the risk of developing lung cancer among Florida women who had never smoked cigarettes. They reported a strong protective effect associated with total vegetable consumption and for intake of carotene. The odds ratio for the highest quartile compared to lowest of vegetable consumption was 0.2, and the odds ratios for total and beta-carotene consumption were 0.3 and 0.4, respectively. Retinol intake was not associated with a decreased risk of lung cancer, and while there was an inverse association of risk with vitamin C intake, it was nonsignificant.[73]

V. GENERAL CONCLUSIONS, SUMMARY, AND IMPLICATIONS

It appears that women are more susceptible to the carcinogenic effects of tobacco smoke, as well as those in environmental tobacco smoke. They may also be more susceptible to DNA damage from nontobacco-related environmental sources such as radon, asbestos, and polycyclic aromatic hydrocarbons. For whatever reasons this increased susceptibility might occur, whether it be due to decreased clearance of nicotine, gender differences in metabolism of carcinogens, or the influence of estrogen on all of the above, women appear to be at greater risk than men, given equal carcinogenic exposures.

In terms of dietary factors and lung cancer risk in women, the data do not support a link between lung cancer risk and cholesterol or fat intakes. Fruit and vegetable consumption appears to be protective, at least in those few studies which specifically targeted women with lung cancer. For those women who were nonsmokers, increased consumption of raw fruits and vegetables decreased passive smoking risk. Interestingly, in assessing diet and lung cancer survival, increased consumption of vegetables and fruit was seen as protective in women, but not in men.

The beta-carotene story is an object lesson in how we need to be cautious in applying specific nutrient interventions in the real world outside the laboratory. Although we see in many studies the benefits of fruit and vegetable consumption, to single out only one nutrient has not proven wise.

Future research in the area of diet and lung cancer prevention should most likely focus on the effects of a diet rich in fruits and vegetables as an intervention in women only, since the data appear to be more compelling in that gender group. Also, more research into what gender differences exist in carcinogen metabolism and how that might be modulated by diet should also be pursued. Finally, although it appears obvious, smoking cessation programs targeted specifically toward women smokers, as well as nonsmoking women married to smokers, would also address much of the causation of women's lung cancers.

REFERENCES

1. Parker, S.L., Tong, T., Bolden, S., and Wingo, P.A., Cancer statistics 1997, *CA Cancer J. Clin.*, 47, 5, 1997.
2. Yesner, R., Sobin, L., Shimosato, Y., and Spencer, H., Eds., *International Histological Classification of Tumors*, Vol. 1, 2nd ed., World Health Organization, Geneva, 1982.
3. Mackay, B., Lukeman, J.M., and Ordonez, N.G., *Tumors of the Lung*, W.B. Saunders, Philadelphia, 1991.

4. Churg, A., Tumors of the lung, in *Pathology of the Lung*, Thurlbeck, W., Ed., Thieme Medical Publishers, New York, 1988, 311.

5. Mountain, C., Lung cancer staging classification, *Clin. Chest Med.*, 14, 43, 1993.

6. Cotran, R.S., Kumar, V., and Robbins, S.L., *Robbins Pathologic Basis of Disease*, 5th ed., W.B. Saunders, Philadelphia, 1994, chap. 15.

7. Carbone, D.P. and Minna, J.D., The molecular genetics of lung cancer, *Adv. Intern. Med.*, 37, 153, 1992.

8. Slebos, R.J., Kibbelaar, R.E., Dalesio, O., Stom, J., Meijer, C.J., Wagenaar, S.S., Vanderschueren, R.G., van Zandwijk, N., Mooi, W.J., Bos, J.L., and Rodenhuis, S., K-*ras* oncogene activation as a prognostic marker in adenocarcinoma of the lung, *New Engl. J. Med.*, 323, 561, 1990.

9. Johnson, B., Ihde, D., Makuch, R.W., Gazdar, A.F., Carney, D.N., Oie, H., Russell, E., Nau, M.M., and Minna, J.D., *myc* family oncogene amplification in tumor cell lines established from small cell lung cancer patients and its relationship to clinical status and course, *J. Clin. Invest.*, 79, 1629, 1987.

10. Takahashi, T., Obata, Y., Sekido, Y., Hida, T., Ueda, R., Watanabe, H., Ariyoshi, Y., Sugira, T., and Takahashi, T., Expression and amplification of *myc* gene family in small cell lung cancer and its relation to biological characteristics, *Cancer Res.*, 49, 2683, 1989.

11. Slebos, R., Evers, S., Wagenaar, S.S., and Rodenhuis, S., Cellular protooncogenes are infrequently amplified in untreated non-small cell lung cancer, *Br. J. Cancer*, 59, 76, 1989.

12. Harbour, J.W., Lai, S.L., Whang-Peng, J., Gazdar, A.F., Minna, J.F., and Kaye, F.J., Abnormalities in structure and expression of the human retinoblastoma gene in SCLC, *Science*, 241, 353, 1988.

13. Takahashi, T., Nau, M., Chiba, I., Birrer, M.J., Rosenberg, R.K., Vincour, M., Levitt, M., Pass, H., Gazdar, A.F., and Minna, J.D., *p53*: a frequent target for genetic abnormalities in lung cancer, *Science*, 246, 491, 1989.

14. Chiba, I., Takahashi, T., Nau, M., D'Aminco, D., Curiel, D.T., Mitsudomi, T., Buchhagen, D.L., Carbone, D., Piantadosi, S., Koga, H., Reissman, P.T., Slamon, D.J., Holmes, E.C., and Minna, J.D., Mutations in the *p53* gene are frequent in primary, resected non-small cell lung cancer, *Oncogene*, 5, 1603, 1990.

15. Kratzke, R.A., Schimizu, E., and Kaye, F.J., Oncogenes in human lung cancer, in *Oncogenes and Tumor Suppressor Genes in Human Malignancies*, Benz, C.C. and Liu, E.T., Eds., Kluwer Academic Publishers, Boston, 1993, 61.

16. Kao-Shan, C.S., Fine, R.L., Whang-Peng, J., Lee, E.C., and Chabner, B.A., Increased fragile sites and sister chromatid exchanges in bone marrow and peripheral blood of young cigarette smokers, *Cancer Res.*, 47, 6278, 1987.

17. Ooi, W.L., Elston, R.C., Chen, V.W., Bailey-Wilson, J.E., and Rothschild, H., Increased familial risk for lung cancer, *J. Natl. Cancer Inst.*, 76, 217, 1986.

18. Caporaso, N., Hayes, R.B., Dosemeci, M., Hoover, R., Ayesh, R., Hetzel, M., and Idle, J., Lung cancer risk, occupational exposure, and the debrisoquine metabolic phenotype, *Cancer Res.*, 49, 3675, 1989.

19. McLemore, T.L., Adelberg, S., Czerwinski, M., Hubbard, W.C., Yu, S.J., Storeng, R., Wood, T.G., Hines, R.N., and Boyd, M.R., Altered regulation of the cytochrome P4501A1 gene expression in pulmonary carcinoma cell lines, *J. Natl. Cancer Inst.*, 81, 1787, 1989.

20. Hirvonen, A., Husgafvel-Puisiainen, K., Anttila, S., and Vainio, H., The *GSTM1* null phenotype as a potential risk modifier for squamous cell carcinoma of the lung, *Carcinogenesis*, 14, 1479, 1993.

21. Blot, W.J. and Fraumeni, J.F., Jr., Cancers of the lung and pleura, in *Cancer Epidemiology and Prevention*, 2nd ed., Schottenfeld, D. and Fraumeni, J.F., Jr., Eds., Oxford University Press, New York, 1996, chap. 31.

22. Ernster, V.L., The epidemiology of lung cancer in women, *Ann. Epidemiol.*, 4, 102, 1994.

23. Environmental Protection Agency, Respiratory Health Effects of Passive Smoking: Lung Cancer and Other Disorders, EPA/600/6-90/006F, Office of Research and Development, EPA, Washington, D.C., December 1992.

24. Gao, Y.T., Blot, W.J., Zheng, W., Ershow, A.G., Hsu, C.W., Levin, L.I., Zhang, R., and Fraumeni, J.F., Jr., Lung cancer among Chinese women, *Int. J. Cancer*, 40, 604, 1987.

25. Mumford, J.L., He, X.Z., Chapman, R.S., Cao, S.R., Harris, D.B., Li, X.M., Xian, Y.L., Jiang, W.Z., Xu, C.W., Chuang, J.C., Wilson, W.E., and Cooke, M., Lung cancer and indoor pollution in Xuan Wei, China, *Science*, 235, 217, 1987.

26. Anon., Cancer incidence trends in U.S. women, *J. Natl. Cancer Inst.*, 88, 1806, 1996.

27. Jenks, S., Gender may render women at risk for lung cancer, *J. Natl. Cancer Inst.*, 88, 144, 1996.

28. American Cancer Society, *Cancer Facts and Figures—1994*, Atlanta, American Cancer Society, 1994.

29. Zang, E.A. and Wynder, E.L., Differences in lung cancer risk between men and women: examination of the evidence, *J. Natl. Cancer Inst.*, 88, 183, 1996.

30. Brownson, R.C., Chang, J.C., and Davis, J.R., Gender and histologic type variations in smoking-related risk of lung cancer, *Epidemiology*, 3, 61, 1992.

31. Risch, H.A., Howe, G.R., Jain, M., Burch, D.J., Holloway, E.J., and Miller, A.B., Are female smokers at higher risk for lung cancer than male smokers? A case-control analysis by histologic type, *Am. J. Epidemiol.*, 138, 281, 1993.

32. Osann, K.E., Anton-Culver, H., Kurosaki, T., and Taylor, T., Sex differences in lung cancer risk associated with cigarette smoking, *Int. J. Cancer*, 54, 44, 1993.

33. Dwyer, T., Blizzard, L., Shugg, D., Hill, D., and Ansari, M.Z., Higher lung cancer rates in young women than in young men: Tasmania, 1983–1992, *Cancer Causes Control*, 5, 351, 1994.

34. Cohn, B.A., Wingard, D.L., Cirillo, P.M., Cohen, R.D., Reynolds, P., and Kaplan, G.A., Re: differences in lung cancer risk between men and women: examination of the evidence, *J. Natl. Cancer Inst.*, 88, 1867, 1996.

35. Beckett, A.H., Gorrod, J.W., and Jenner, P., The effect of smoking on nicotine metabolism *in vivo* in man, *J. Pharm. Pharmacol.* (Suppl.), 62S, 1971.

36. Benowitz, N.L. and Jacob, P., III, Daily intake of nicotine during cigarette smoking, *Clin. Pharmacol. Ther.*, 35, 499, 1984.

37. Klein, A.E. and Gorrod, J.W., Age as a factor in the metabolism of nicotine, *Eur. J. Drug Metab. Pharmacol.*, 1, 51, 1978.

38. Kato, R., Sex-related differences in drug metabolism, *Drug Metab. Rev.*, 3, 1, 1974.

39. Jain, M., Burch, J.D., Howe, G.R., and Miller, A.B., Dietary factors and risk of lung cancer: results from a case-control study, Toronto, 1981–1985, *Int. J. Cancer*, 45, 287, 1990.

40. Byers, T.E., Graham, S., Haughey, B.P., Marshall, J.R., and Swanson, M.K., Diet and lung cancer risk: findings from the western New York study, *Am. J. Epidemiol.*, 125, 351, 1987.

41. Hinds, M.W., Kolonel, L.N., Hankin, J.H., and Lee, J., Dietary cholesterol and lung cancer risk in a multiethnic population in Hawaii, *Int. J. Cancer*, 32, 727, 1983.

42. Goodman, M.T., Kolonel, L.N., Yoshizawa, C.N., and Hankin, J.H., The effect of dietary cholesterol and fat on the risk of lung cancer in Hawaii, *Am. J. Epidemiol.*, 128, 1241, 1988.

43. Alvanja, M.C., Brown, C.C., Swanson, C., and Brownson, R.C., Saturated fat intake and lung cancer risk among nonsmoking women in Missouri, *J. Natl. Cancer Inst.*, 85, 1906, 1993.

44. Shekelle, R.B., Rossof, A.H., and Stamler, J., Dietary cholesterol and incidence of lung cancer: the Western Electric Study, *Am. J. Epidemiol.*, 134, 480, 1991.

45. Knekt, P., Seppanen, R., Jarvinen, R., Virtamo, J., Hyvonen, L., Pukkala, E., and Teppo, L., Dietary cholesterol, fatty acids, and the risk of lung cancer among men, *Nutr. Cancer*, 16, 267, 1991.

46. Heilbrun, L.K., Nomura, A.M., and Stemmermann, G.N., Dietary cholesterol and lung cancer risk among Japanese men in Hawaii, *Am. J. Clin. Nutr.*, 39, 375, 1984.

47. Wu, Y., Zheng, W., Sellers, T.A., Kushi, L., Bostick, R.M., and Potter, J.D., Dietary cholesterol, fat, and lung cancer incidence among older women: the Iowa Women's Health Study (United States), *Cancer Causes Control*, 5, 395, 1994.

48. Maclennan, R., Ca Costa, J., Day, N.E., Law, C.H., Ng, Y.K., and Shammugaratnam, K., Risk factors for lung cancer in Singapore Chinese, a population with high female incidence rates, *Int. J. Cancer*, 20, 854, 1997.

49. Mettlin, C., Graham, S., and Swanson, M., Vitamin A and cancer, *J. Natl. Cancer Inst.*, 62, 1435, 1979.

50. Ziegler, R.G., Mason, T.J., Stemhagen, A., Hoover, R., Schoenberg, J.B., Gridley, G., Virgo, P.W., and Fraumeni, J.F., Jr., Carotenoid intake, vegetables, and the risk of lung cancer among white men in New Jersey, *Am. J. Epidemiol.*, 123, 1080, 1986.

51. Pisani, P., Berrino, F., Macaluso, M., Pastorino, U., Crosignani, P., and Baldasseroni, A., Carrots, green vegetables, and lung cancer: a case-control study, *Int. J. Epidemiol.*, 15, 463, 1986.

52. Koo, L.C., Dietary habits and lung cancer risk among Chinese females in Hong Kong who never smoked, *Nutr. Cancer*, 11, 155, 1988.

53. Fontham, E.T.H., Pickle, L.W., Haensel, W., Correa, P., Lin, Y., and Falk, R., Dietary vitamin A and C and lung cancer risk in Louisiana, *Cancer*, 62, 2267, 1988.

54. Le Marchand, L., Yoshizawa, C.N., Kolonel, L.N., Hankin, J.H., and Goodman, M.T., Vegetable consumption and lung cancer risk: a population-based case-control study in Hawaii, *J. Natl. Cancer Inst.*, 81, 1158, 1989.

55. Mettlin, C., Milk drinking, other beverage habits, and lung cancer risk, *Int. J. Cancer*, 43, 608, 1989.

56. Forman, M.R., Yao, S.X., Graubard, B.I., Qiao, Y.L., McAdams, M., and Taylor, P.R., The effect of dietary intake of fruits and vegetables in the odds ratios of lung cancer among Yunnan tin miners (abstract), *Am. J. Epidemiol.*, 134, 725, 1991.

57. Kalandidi, A., Katsouyanni, K., Voropoupou, N., Bastas, G., Saracci, R., and Trichopoulos, D., Passive smoking, and diet in the etiology of lung cancer among nonsmokers, *Cancer Causes Control*, 1, 15, 1990.

58. Swanson, C.A., Mao, B.L., Li, J.Y., Lubin, J.H., Yao, S.X., Wang, J.Z., Cai, S.K., Hou, Y., Luo, Q.S., and Blot, W.J., Dietary determinants of lung-cancer risk: results from a case-control study in Yunnan Province, China, *Int. J. Cancer*, 50, 876, 1992.

59. Kvale, G., Bjelke, E., and Gart, J.J., Dietary habits and lung cancer risk, *Int. J. Cancer*, 31, 397, 1983.

60. Long-de, W. and Hammond, E.C., Lung cancer, fruit, green salad, and vitamin pills, *Chin. Med. J.* (Engl. ed.), 98, 206, 1985.

61. Frase, G.E., Beeson, W.L., and Phillips, R.L., Diet and lung cancer in California Seventh-Day Adventists, *Am. J. Epidemiol.*, 133, 683, 1991.

62. Ferguson, M.K., Skosey, C., Hoffman, P.C., and Golomb, H.M., Sex-associated differences in presentation and survival in patients with lung cancer, *J. Clin. Oncol.*, 8, 1402, 1990.

63. McDuffie, H.H., Klaasen, D.J., and Dosman, J.A., Female–male differences in patients with primary lung cancer, *Cancer*, 59, 1825, 1987.

64. Steinmetz, K.A., Potter, J.D., and Folsom, A.R., Vegetables, fruit, and lung cancer in the Iowa Women's Health Study, *Cancer Res.*, 53, 536, 1993.

65. Matonoski, G., Kanchanaraksa, S., Lantry, D., and Chang, Y., Characteristics of nonsmoking women in NHANES I and NHANES I epidemiologic follow-up study with exposures to spouses who smoke, *Am. J. Epidemiol.*, 142, 149, 1995.

66. Mayne, S.T., Janerick, D.T., Greenwald, P., Chorost, S., Tucci, C., Zaman, M.B., Melamed, M.R., Kiely, M., and McKneally, M.F., Dietary beta-carotene and lung cancer risk in the United States, *J. Natl. Cancer Inst.*, 86, 33, 1994.

67. Goodman, M.T., Kolonel, L.N., Wilkens, L.R., Yoshizawa, C.N., Le Marchand, L., and Hankin, J.H., Dietary factors in lung cancer prognosis, *Eur. J. Cancer*, 28, 495, 1992.

68. The Alpha-Tocopherol, Beta-Carotene Cancer Prevention Study Group, The effect of vitamin E and beta-carotene on the incidence of lung cancer and other cancers in male smokers, *New Engl. J. Med.*, 330, 1029, 1994.

69. Omenn, G.S., Goodman, G.E., Thornquist, M.D., Balmes, J., Cullen, M.R., Glass, A., Keogh, J.P., Meyskens, F.L., Valamis, B., Williams, J.H., Barnhart, S., and Hammar, S., Effects of a combination of beta-carotene and vitamin A on lung cancer and cardiovascular disease, *New Engl. J. Med.*, 334, 1150, 1996.

70. Smigel, K., Beta-carotene fails to prevent cancer in two major studies: CARET intervention stopped, *J. Natl. Cancer Inst.*, 88, 145, 1996.

71. Hennekens, C.H., Buring, J.E., Manson, J.E., Stampfer, M., Rosner, B., Cook, N.R., Belanger, C., LaMotte, F., Gaziano, J.M., Ridker, P.M., Willett, W., and Peto, R., Lack of effect of long-term supplementation with beta-carotene on the

incidence of malignant neoplasms and cardiovascular disease, *New Engl. J. Med.*, 334, 1145, 1996.

72. Wu-Williams, A.H., Dai, X.D., Blot, W., Xu, Z.Y., Sun, X.W., Xiao, H.P., Stone, B.J., Yu, S.F., Feng, Y.P., Ershow, A.G., Sun, J., Fraumeni, J.F., Jr., and Henderson, B.E., Lung cancer among women in northeast China, *Br. J. Cancer*, 62, 982, 1990.

73. Candelora, E.C., Stockwell, H.G., Armstrong, A.W., and Pinkham, P.A., Dietary intake and risk of lung cancer in women who never smoked, *Nutr. Cancer*, 17, 263, 1992.

CHAPTER 8

WOMEN'S CANCER POLICY ISSUES AND CURRENT TRIALS

CONTENTS

I. NATIONAL OFFICE OF WOMEN'S HEALTH

Women's health research has become a major endeavor of the National Institutes of Health (NIH) and the U.S. Public Health Service (USPHS). Historically, women had apparently been left out of the equation in organized medicine and public health prior to the early 1980s. The practice of medicine was a male-dominated profession, and as such, women had been conspicuously left out of clinical trials. Even experimental research had used predominantly male animals due to possible confounding of results by a cyclical hormonal milieu. In order "to assess the problems of women's health in the context of the lives women in American lead today," the Assistant Secretary for Health, Dr. Edward N. Brandt, Jr., appointed a USPHS Task Force on Women's Health Issues in 1983.[1] Recommendations of that task force were organized to include:[2]

1. Promotion of a safe, healthful physical and social environment
2. Provision of services for prevention and treatment of disease
3. Research and evaluation
4. Recruitment and training of healthcare personnel
5. Public education and dissemination of research information
6. Design of guidelines for legislative and regulatory measures

From the guidelines on research and evaluation, there were three major recommendations made by the task force:[2]

1. Expansion of biomedical and behavioral research with an emphasis on conditions and diseases unique to or more prevalent in women in all age groups
2. Expansion of research and development for more effective, acceptable, and safe contraceptive methods for both men and women
3. Expansion of studies of causes, prevention, improved diagnosis, and treatment of debilitating diseases such as breast and other reproductive system cancers, sexually transmitted diseases, arthritides including lupus, osteoporosis, and certain mental disorders

This last recommendation has significantly impacted the area of research into women's cancers and is one that we shall focus on in terms of national multicenter clinical trials.

Following the publication of the task force's recommendations report, a National Conference on Women's Health was held in June 1986, which was sponsored by the USPHS Coordinating Committee on Women's Health Issues and the Food and Drug Administration.[3] Two of the issues discussed at the conference were nutrition and cancer, with a focus on the health of women. The USPHS Task Force's recommendations also included the establishment of groups within each agency to implement the recommendations according to their appropriate responsibilities.[1] The NIH Advisory Committee on Women's Health Issues was established in 1985 and, among other issues, has specifically identified the limited inclusion of women in clinical trials and then recommended policies to correct this shortage. This policy has received further support from Congress in the formation of a Women's Health Caucus and in their request of the Government Accounting Office (GAO) to address the inclusion of women in clinical trials.[1] The report of the GAO was presented in June 1990, and the NIH reemphasized its policy that requires research grant applicants to justify exclusion or underrepresentation of women in clinical trials.[1]

In September 1990, the acting director of the NIH announced the creation of the Office of Research on Women's Health (ORWH). The ORWH is charged with assuring that research conducted and supported by NIH adequately addresses issues regarding women's health and that there is appropriate participation of women in clinical research, especially in clinical trials.[1] There are three main goals for this office:

1. To strengthen and enhance NIH efforts to improve prevention, diagnosis, and treatment of illness in women
2. To assure that research conducted and supported by NIH addresses issues regarding women's health appropriately
3. To assure that there is appropriate participation of women in clinical studies

One of ORWH's first accomplishments was a 1992 report that served as a basis for its research agenda; its recommendations focus on scientific issues affecting women's health from birth to old age.[4] To implement these recommendations, the ORWH does not fund studies directly, but instead provides funds through NIH institutes and centers to augment new research initiatives, to expand ongoing studies to address high-priority areas concerning women's health, and to expand the participation of women in clinical studies.[4] As such, the ORWH is playing a key advisory role in NIH's Women's Health Initiative, which is the largest clinical trial ever undertaken by the NIH with men and/or women.

II. PREVIOUS LARGE STUDIES OF WOMEN'S DIET AND CANCER

A. Nurses' Health Study

Most of the previous large studies of issues related to women's diet and cancer have been cohort studies involving large numbers of women who are followed for a period of time to determine the outcome of incident cancers. Most notable of this type of study is the Nurses' Health Study, which has gathered data on the diets of 98,464 women and followed them since 1980,[5] and the Iowa Women's Health Study.[6] The Nurses' Health Study cohort was defined in 1976 when 121,700 female registered nurses 30–55 years of age who were living in 11 large U.S. states completed a mailed questionnaire on known and suspected risk factors for cancer and coronary heart disease.[5] Every 2 years, follow-up questionnaires have been sent to update information on potential risk factors and identify new cases of cancer and other diseases. In 1980, the questionnaires were expanded to include an assessment of diet. After four mailings, 98,464 women returned the 1980 dietary questionnaire,[5] and after certain exclusions for incomplete questionnaires or history of diseases affecting eating behavior, the final baseline population for dietary assessment was 88,751.[5]

B. Iowa Women's Health Study

The Iowa Women's Health Study was a prospective study of Iowa women comprising the second largest cohort examined.[6] In 1986, 98,030 women age 55–69 years who had a valid Iowa driver's license in 1985 were selected randomly and mailed a questionnaire on known and suspected cancer risk factors.[6] There were 41,837 respondents with a mean age of 61.7 years; 99% were white, 39% had education beyond high school, 19% had less than a high school education, and 34% resided in cities with populations of 10,000 or greater, with 27% living in rural areas.[6] The dietary questionnaires and statistical analyses were similar between the Nurses' Health Study and the Iowa Women's Health Study.

III. CLINICAL INTERVENTION TRIALS IN WOMEN'S CANCERS

A. The Women's Health Initiative

The Women's Health Initiative (WHI) is the largest clinical trial ever undertaken by the NIH. This is a $625-million 15-year study of 63,000 women that will address major causes of morbidity and mortality in postmenopausal women. A parallel observational study will follow a cohort of 100,000 women over 9 years to help predict who will develop coronary heart disease, breast or colorectal cancer, and fractures and who will die as a result of these diseases. The WHI began recruiting test subjects in 15 vanguard clinical centers across the country in 1993, and with the addition of another 29 centers in 1994 will attempt to enroll over 160,000 postmenopausal women between the ages of 50 and 79.[7] The WHI will focus on breast and colorectal cancers, coronary heart disease, and osteoporosis and will assess the value of dietary patterns, hormone replacement therapy (HRT), and calcium plus vitamin D supplementation in preventing these conditions.[7] The WHI consists of three components: a controlled clinical trial (blinded to the fullest extent possible), a companion prospective observational study to identify predictors of disease, and a study of community approaches to encourage women to adopt healthful behaviors.[7]

The clinical trial will enroll 63,000 women who will be randomized to treatment or control arms after choosing to receive one or more of the three interventions: a low-fat diet, HRT, or calcium/vitamin D supplementation. The trial proposes to address the following specific questions:[7] (1) Does a low-fat dietary pattern prevent breast cancer, colorectal cancer, and coronary heart disease? (2) Does HRT with estrogen alone or estrogen plus progestin prevent coronary heart disease and osteoporosis? and (3) Does calcium plus vitamin D supplementation prevent osteoporotic fractures and colorectal cancer? For each of these questions, the overall question will be whether the benefits outweigh the risks associated with each intervention. The study design for the WHI is shown in Figure 8.1.[8]

Since this book is primarily about women's cancers, we will specifically address the diet modification arm of the WHI. The primary outcome of this arm

WOMEN'S HEALTH INITIATIVE

Arm/#	Treatment/#	Primary Endpoints (Secondary Endpoints)
I. HRT/32,000		
Have uterus	ERT/30%	Coronary disease
	PERT/28%	(cancer, osteoporosis)
	Placebo/42%	
No uterus	ERT/58%	
	Placebo/42%	
II. Diet Modification/48,000		
	20% fat diet/40%	Breast, colorectal cancer
	Usual diet/60%	(coronary disease)
III. Calcium + Vitamin D/45,000		
	Calcium + vitamin D/50%	Osteoporosis
	Placebo/50%	(colorectal cancer)

Figure 8.1   Study design of the Women's Health Initiative clinical trial (adapted from Assaf and Carleton[8]).

is breast and colorectal cancer. The women will be randomly allocated to their usual diet or to an intervention diet with 20% or fewer calories from fat.[7] Previous smaller studies such as the Women's Health Trial[9] and others[10] demonstrated that low-fat diets could be maintained in a study population. An ancillary goal of the WHI is to reduce saturated fat calories to less than 7% of all calories. Compensatory changes in the diet will also include increases in complex carbohydrates, fruits, vegetables, and grain products. The nutritional adequacy of the diet will be monitored with food frequency questionnaires throughout the trial:[7] 48,000 women will be enrolled in this arm, and it is projected from the power calculation that even small reductions in breast and colorectal cancers, as well as heart disease, will be detectable.[7]

The observational study will enroll about 100,000 additional women who will be involved in assessment of the risk factors and outcomes associated with health and diseases peculiar to women. One of the questions that will be asked is whether women have different risk factors than men for common chronic diseases.[7] Since the extensive epidemiological database on cardiovascular disease has been derived from studies that relate mostly to men, such as the Framingham Study, MRFIT, and the Seven Countries Study,[7] the inclusion of cardiovascular disease as an outcome seems appropriate for the WHI. Although the Nurses' Health Study gave us a significant database on the health of women, there are still many gaps in knowledge.

The community trials part of the WHI has as its purpose the evaluation of strategies to achieve healthful behaviors, including improved diet, nutritional supplementation, smoking prevention and cessation, increased physical activity, and early disease detection for women of all races, ethnic groups, and socioeconomic strata.[11] Although this is a laudable goal, the exact plan for this part of the study remains poorly defined, although the community prevention trials are meant to instruct low-income and ethnic groups in healthy lifestyles.

Although the WHI sounds like the answer to many serious questions in the women's health arena, it has not been without its detractors. A special panel at the Institute of Medicine issued a very critical review of the WHI just as it was beginning to accrue subjects in the fall of 1993.[11] The panel had harsh comments about the feasibility of the trial, especially that the trial is unlikely to stay within budget or find solid evidence linking low-fat diets to a reduction in breast cancer rates.[11] Lynn Rosenberg, an epidemiologist and member of the review panel, stated that "it's a very weak hypothesis that changing the diets of women in their fifties, sixties, or seventies will influence their risks of getting breast cancer."[11]

B. The Harvard Women's Health Study

The Harvard Women's Health Study (WHS) is a double-blind, placebo-controlled, randomized trial designed to evaluate the risks and benefits of low-dose aspirin, as well as the antioxidant vitamins beta-carotene and vitamin E, in the primary prevention of cardiovascular disease and cancer. Vitamin E will be given at 600 IU on alternate days, supplied by the Natural Source Vitamin E Association, and low-dose aspirin will be given at 100 mg on alternate days, to be supplied by Miles, Inc. This trial, begun in 1992, will also involve interventions in healthy postmenopausal women in the United States and plans to enroll 40,000 female health professionals with no previous history of either cardiovascular disease or cancer.[12] The design of the WHS is analogous to the Physicians' Health Study, which began in 1982 and is still ongoing.[13] The design of the randomization scheme is presented in Figure 8.2.[12] The WHS will be conducted entirely by mail, with the study agents provided in convenient monthly calendar packs to aid in compliance.[12] Because of this, it will be one of the least expensive primary prevention trials ever conducted with women.

C. The Women's Intervention Nutrition Study

Finally, in terms of nutrition interventions and prevention of women's cancers, we must mention the Women's Intervention Nutrition Study (WINS),[14]

Women's Health Study
40,000+ Postmenopausal Women Health Professionals

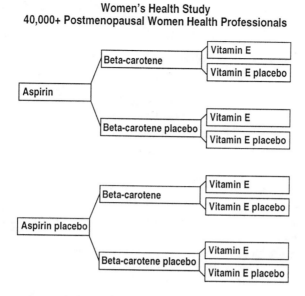

Figure 8.2 Study design of the Harvard Women's Health Study (adapted from Buring and Hennekens[12]).

the goal of which is to reduce total fat intake to 15% of total calories among postmenopausal women with stage I or stage II breast cancer who have already had standard therapy. This is a multi-institutional clinical trial to test the effects of a low-fat diet in breast cancer patients with histologically positive or negative axillary nodes and will examine adherence to a dietary modification program in conjunction with adjuvant chemotherapy or hormonal therapy. The primary objective of this study is to assess the feasibility of patients' adherence to the dietary modifications. Secondary objectives will include identification of a set of behavioral and psychosocial variables that can be used as predictors of dietary change. This study is considered a critical intermediate step in the decision process for determination of whether to conduct a full-scale outcome study to evaluate dietary modification as an adjunct to standard breast cancer therapy.[15]

D. Summary and Conclusions

As can be seen by the NIH commitment to these immense clinical trials conducted only with women, we have indeed come a long way toward medical equality. However, these trials are lengthy and expensive and require enormous effort on the part of participants and researchers. The benefits to be achieved from these efforts could be substantial, and if definitive answers are discovered, then the burden of heart disease, osteoporosis, and cancers of several sites in women could be more effectively prevented. It is our sincere hope that these efforts will be beneficial to the entire population and increase our understanding of the critical role of diet in chronic disease.

REFERENCES

1. Cummings, N.B., Women's health and nutrition research: U.S. governmental concerns, *J. Am. Coll. Nutr.*, 12, 329, 1993.
2. Women's Health, Report of the Public Health Service Task Force on Women's Health Issues, Vol. I, U.S. Government Printing Office, Washington, D.C., 1985, 100: 73–106.
3. Women's health, *J. U.S. Public Health Service*, July–August (Suppl.), 1986.
4. Pinn, V.W., The role of the NIH's Office of Research on Women's Health, *Acad. Med.*, 9, 698, 1994.
5. Willett, W.C., Stampfer, M.J., Colditz, G.A., Rosner, B.A., and Speizer, F.E., Relation of meat, fat, and fiber intake to the risk of colon cancer in a prospective study among women, *New Engl. J. Med.*, 323, 1664, 1990.
6. Bostick, R.M., Potter, J.D., Steinmetz, K.A., Kushi, L.H., Sellars, T.A., McKenzie, D.R., Gapstur, S.M., and Folsom, A.R., Sugar, meat, and fat intake and non-dietary risk factors for colon cancer incidence in Iowa women (United States), *Cancer Causes Control*, 5, 38, 1994.
7. Kirchstein, R., Largest clinical trial ever gets underway, *J. Am. Med. Assoc.*, 270, 1521, 1993.
8. Assaf, A.R. and Carleton, R.A., The Women's Health Initiative clinical trial and observational study: history and overview, *Rhode Island Med.*, 77, 424, 1994.
9. White, E., Shattuck, A.L., Kristal, A.R., Urban, N., Prentice, R.L., Henderson, M.M., Insull, W., Jr., Moskowitz, M., Goldman, S., and Woods, M.N., Maintenance of a low-fat diet: follow-up of the Women's Health Trial, *Cancer Epidemiol. Biomarkers Prev.*, 1, 315, 1992.
10. Simon, M.S., Heilbrun, L.K., Boomer, A., Kresge, C., Depper, J., Kim, P.N., Valeriote, F., and Martino, S., A randomized trial of a low-fat dietary intervention in women at high risk for breast cancer, *Nutr. Cancer*, 27, 136, 1997.
11. Marshall, E., Women's Health Initiative draws flak, *Science*, 262, 838, 1993.
12. Buring, J.E. and Hennekens, C.H., The Women's Health Study: summary of the study design, *J. Myocard. Ischemia*, 4, 27, 1992.
13. The Steering Committee for the Physicians' Health Study Research Group, Final report on the aspirin component of the ongoing Physicians' Health Study, *New Engl. J. Med.*, 321, 121, 1989.
14. Chlebowski, R.T., Blackburn, G.L., Buzzard, I.M., Rose, D.P., Martino, S., Khandekar, J.D., et al., Adherence to a dietary fat intake reduction program in postmenopausal women receiving therapy for early breast cancer: the Women's Intervention Nutrition Study, *J. Clin. Oncol.*, 11, 2072, 1993.
15. Greenwald, P. and Clifford, C., Dietary prevention, in *Cancer Prevention and Control*, Greenwald, P., Kramer, B.S., and Weed, D.L., Eds., Marcel Dekker, New York, 1995, chap. 18.

CHAPTER 9

SUMMARY, CONCLUSIONS, AND DIRECTIONS FOR FUTURE RESEARCH

CONTENTS

I. GENERAL SUMMARY AND CONCLUSIONS

A. *Healthy People 2000* Goals

In 1990, the U.S. Department of Health and Human Services published *Healthy People 2000*, which set goals for all Americans, including increasing the span of healthy life, reducing health disparities, and achieving access to preventive services.[1] Progress toward those goals was recently reviewed, and progress was reported as a percentage of the target achieved. In the area of women's cancers, the *Healthy People 2000* objectives had focused on screening for breast and cervical cancer and reducing mortality from those diseases.[2] The cancer-related objectives for the year 2000 for women's cancers were:

1. Reduce breast cancer deaths to no more than 20.6 per 100,000 women per year (1987 baseline 23.0 per 100,000); 63% of target achieved
2. Reduce cervical cancer deaths to no more than 1.3 per 100,000 women per year (1987 baseline 2.8 per 100,000); 13% of target achieved
3. Increase to at least 60% the proportion of women 50 years and older who have received a clinical breast exam and mammogram in the past 2 years (1987 baseline 25%); 89% of target achieved
4. Increase to at least 95% the proportion of women 18 years and older who have ever received a Pap test (1987 baseline 88%); 86% of target achieved
5. Increase to at least 85% the proportion of women who have received a Pap test in the past 3 years (1987 baseline 75%); 20% of target achieved
6. Ensure that mammograms meet quality standards through American College of Radiology inspection and certification of 100% of mammography facilities according to the requirements of the Mammography Quality Standards Act (1990 baseline 19%); 56% of target achieved

This recent review demonstrates that where screening programs for breast cancer are concerned, the year 2000 goal is close to being realized. For Pap tests, the objective falls seriously short of achievement. But the most important statistics for our purposes in this book are the goals for reducing the death rates for breast and cervical cancer in U.S. women. Although screening is an important part of reducing the death rate, primary prevention, potentially through nutrition and other lifestyle changes, may have its greatest impact here. For each cancer of women that we have focused on in this book, we would like to summarize the findings and perhaps offer some recommendations.

B. Summary of Recommendations for Specific Women's Cancers

1. Breast Cancer

Breast cancer risk factors have been more extensively studied than those for any other cancer that occurs in women. In general, reproductive factors such as age at menarche, age at menopause, pregnancy, lactation, and menstrual cycle length seem to be major determinants of breast cancer probability. In addition, family history has also been a strong predictor of risk, especially in those women carrying germline mutations in the *BRCA* genes for susceptibility.

Although the genetic link predominates in only about 10% of breast cancers, there is still much we need to know about the function of the *BRCA* genes and how they interact with environmental factors such as cigarette smoking, hormone replacement therapy (HRT) use, and dietary practices. For the vast majority of women diagnosed with breast cancer, the etiology of their cancer remains completely unknown.

Obviously, breast cancer is a hormonally related cancer, and most of the risk factors are mechanistically interpreted through that filter. However, the data on the use of oral contraceptives and HRT do not support a prominent role for exogenous hormones in the etiology of breast cancer, although longer term studies are needed in the case of HRT.

The general conclusions about physical exercise appear to support the idea that increased activity tends to decrease risk. The mechanisms underlying this observation need to be further examined. The issue of cigarette smoking and breast cancer is still inconclusive, with the habit neither substantially decreasing nor increasing risk. However, if one chooses to agree with the Colditz and Frazier[3] model for early intervention to reduce lifetime breast cancer risk, then these two habits emerge as more critical determinants of risk. The message "more exercise and don't smoke" then becomes targeted to adolescent girls rather than postmenopausal women. The adolescent intervention model is intriguing, and more research is needed to validate these ideas.

The controversial link between dietary fat and breast cancer risk has been debated by the best researchers in the diet and cancer field, with no hard conclusions to be drawn. Increased height and weight appear to modestly increase breast cancer risk, as does an increased body mass index, and these variables are presumed to be mechanistically related to higher levels of circulating estrogens in obese postmenopausal women. But a strong compelling association for dietary fat is elusive, possibly due to overlap of variables such as total calories consumed, red meat intake and its cooking preferences (i.e., generation of heterocyclic amines), body mass, and percentage body fat, all of which can be hindered by dietary assessment error bias. Finally, since the underlying cause of breast cancer appears to be related in part to estrogenic exposure, then the relationship between hormone status and dietary fat and associated body mass variables should be more precisely assessed within the same study population. More research is also required into the dietary fat/body mass effects on estrogen metabolism across the life span of the female.

Consumption of the antioxidant vitamins A, E, and C, as well as fruits and vegetables in general, appears to be protective against breast cancer. However, we do not know if there is some property inherent in these specific vitamins which decreases risk or if increased intake is merely a marker for a healthier lifestyle. This concept of the "healthy lifestyle" may be hallmarked by a greater propensity for eating fruits and vegetables and, conversely, lower consumption of dietary fat and meat products and needs further validation. Selenium intake does not appear to modify breast cancer risk, nor does consumption of vitamin D, although both of these nutrients appear to have profound effects at pharmacologic doses in experimental animal studies.

Alcoholic beverage consumption appears to impart a modest increase in risk, although many inconsistencies exist in the data. However, the risk increase may or may not be associated with an increase in estrogenic hormones, and further research in this area is warranted.

The case for phytoestrogens, including soy isoflavones and lignans from flax, is provocative but incomplete. Most work to date has been performed in cell culture or animal models of breast cancer. More extensive data on soy in the diet of Asian women with and without breast cancer would be helpful to sort out whether it is a specific effect of soy or soy intake that is a marker for the lower risk Asian lifestyle.

We still do not know the etiology of human breast cancer beyond that which appears to directly result from *BRCA1* and *BRCA2* mutations. It is possible that two mutagens contained in our foods, such as heterocyclic amines and pesticides, may be involved in the causation of breast cancer. The effects of these potential carcinogens need to be better assessed in future studies, both epidemiological and experimental.

Finally, in light of the fact that the strongest predictor of breast cancer risk still appears to be a family history of the disease, we need to focus future studies of other risk factors, including dietary, on the interaction of environmental risk factors with the hereditary predisposition. Dietary fat may only be a risk determinant in specific high-risk populations, and the protection afforded by fruit and vegetable consumption may also only be effective in the absence of a genetically determined risk. In a future where many women will be tested to identify their risk for breast and other cancers, perhaps studying nutritional factors by risk stratification will yield better clues as to the real role of diet in breast cancer.

2. Cervical Cancer

There is currently overwhelming evidence that infection by human papillomavirus (HPV) is the key risk factor in the development of cervical cancer. Other genetic risk factors predisposing to the disease have only a minor role to play, or they have yet to be identified. Thus, the risk for cervical cancer is more dependent on environmental sexual exposures to HPV than to any predisposing familial susceptibility to this cancer. It is currently unknown whether some individuals are more easily infected with HPV than others in terms of host susceptibility for the virus. Most other factors such as use of oral contraceptives, sexual practices, and infection with other sexually transmitted diseases should all be considered as surrogate variables for promiscuous behavior and, therefore, for increased probability of exposure to and infection with HPV.

The relationship between vitamin A, the carotenoids, and cervical cancer shows some indication that the intake of these nutrients and the overall vitamin A status of the individual may be important in cervical neoplasia, but the large body of data is far from consistent, so no concrete recommendations can be made. Higher intakes of vitamin C may be protective, but the effect may only be evident in women who smoke and, therefore, have higher daily requirements for vitamin C. No conclusions can be drawn for the role of vitamin E in cervical cancer risk.

The case for folate is probably more compelling than for any other nutrient studied in association with cervical cancer. The association between folate status and cervical dysplasia is most convincing, although there are some negative studies. Most interesting is the potential connection between folate status and HPV infection, and more research is needed into the intake of folate and susceptibility to HPV infection following exposure.

In summary, there are no strong compelling nutritional factors which are predictors for cervical cancer, with the possible exception of folate. The overwhelming etiological agent for cervical cancer appears to be HPV infection, which can be somewhat prevented by more prudent sexual practices. However, the area of nutritional modulation of HPV host susceptibility is a research area that needs more attention, as the studies with folate have revealed. There are always permissive host factors to be considered in any viral infection, and that is where nutrition may have its greatest impact in this disease.

3. Ovarian Cancer

The genetic basis of familial ovarian cancer with or without breast involvement has been extensively studied. It appears that hereditary ovarian cancer is causally linked to mutations in *BRCA1,* with a cumulative risk by age 70 of 48%. However, few somatic *BRCA1* mutations have been found in sporadic ovarian tumors. The role of *BRCA2* in ovarian cancer is a lesser one in both hereditary and sporadic tumors. As such, however, these genes account for less than 10% of the cases in the population, so other factors obviously must play a role.

Women's general reproductive functions, such as oral contraceptive use, number of pregnancies, and lactation, appear to be somewhat protective. This is speculated to be due to suppression of ovarian function, which may inhibit the cancer development process for epithelial ovarian cancer.

Studies of obesity, height/weight, and body fat distribution have not shown a consistent association with ovarian cancer risk. Specific dietary items that have been positively associated with ovarian cancer are intake of animal fat and meat products. Vegetable consumption appears to be protective. Two studies reported a link between coffee drinking and risk for ovarian cancer, whereas one did not. Only one recent study has reported a modest increase in risk with alcoholic beverage consumption.

The sum of implications from these studies is, unfortunately, inconclusive. Whereas we can attribute approximately 10% of ovarian cancer cases to mutations in *BRCA1* and *BRCA2*, the vast majority of cases do not have a strong, compelling association with any risk factor, either environmental or dietary. The hormonal influences underlying the development of ovarian cancer need to be better defined, and until we can achieve a better understanding of those mechanisms, the nutritional factors influencing those mechanisms will be poorly understood.

4. Endometrial Cancer

In summarizing the genetic information related to endometrial cancer, it appears that there is some genetic component associated with the cancer, but no target gene for predisposition has been identified. The predominant risk factor for cancer of the uterine corpus appears to be "unopposed" estrogenic stimulation of endometrial tissue, due to either endogenous factors or an endogenous source of the hormones. Whether these endogenous factors are genetically controlled or more environmentally influenced cannot be determined at this time.

The inverse connection between cigarette smoking and endometrial cancer is intriguing, but is not to be considered seriously as an intervention to reduce risk, since the other health risks associated with cigarette smoking far outweigh any potential benefits to be gained. Likewise, there may also be an inverse association between alcoholic beverage consumption and endometrial cancer risk, although these data must be interpreted cautiously as to cause and effect. The hormonal effects of alcohol ingestion on sex hormone binding globulin and serum estrogen levels appear to be beneficial; however, more research is needed into this phenomenon.

Body weight, obesity, body mass index, and body fat distribution all appear to be risk factors for endometrial cancer, and the consensus of the literature cited supports this contention. However, the thought is still that the effects of these variables are ultimately operating through estrogen metabolism and overexposure, still consistent with an "unopposed" estrogen hypothesis. More research is needed on the interactions between hormonal status, these nutritionally related factors, and endometrial cancer risk within the same study population.

Dietary variables such as fat, fruits, and vegetables all seem to point to a trend for increased risk associated with fat intake, meat protein, and total calories in general. There appears to be a role for increased consumption of fruits and vegetables in decreasing risk. However, the data do not point to any specific vitamin as being protective. Again, these conclusions are also consistent with a hormonal hypothesis for endometrial cancer, in that dietary fat may contribute to increased estrogen exposure, either through a direct effect on estrogen metabolism or due to its contribution to obesity.

The implications for reduction of risk for endometrial cancer appear to be inextricably intertwined with hormone status, both endogenous and exogenous. Therefore, it would appear that any future studies of nutritional factors and this cancer should focus on the effects of certain nutrients on hormone status, and case-control studies should attempt to correlate nutrient intake with hormonal status in order to determine a mechanistic link.

5. Lung Cancer

It appears that women are more susceptible to the carcinogenic effects of tobacco smoke, as well as those in environmental tobacco smoke. They may also be more susceptible to DNA damage from nontobacco-related environmental sources, such as radon, asbestos, and polycyclic aromatic hydrocarbons. For whatever reasons this increased susceptibility might occur, whether it be due to decreased clearance of nicotine, gender differences in metabolism of carcinogens, or the influence of estrogen on all of the above, women appear to be at greater risk, given equal exposures.

In terms of dietary factors and lung cancer risk in women, the data do not support a link between lung cancer risk and cholesterol or fat intakes. Fruit and vegetable consumption appears to be protective, at least in those few studies that specifically targeted women with lung cancer. For those women who were nonsmokers, increased consumption of raw fruits and vegetables decreased passive smoking risk. Interestingly, in assessing diet and lung cancer survival, increased consumption of vegetables and fruit was seen as protective in women, but not in men.

The beta-carotene story is an object lesson in how we need to be cautious in applying specific nutrient interventions in the real world outside the laboratory. Although we see in many studies the benefits of fruit and vegetable consumption, to single out only one nutrient has not proven wise.

Future research in the area of diet and lung cancer prevention should most likely focus on the effects of a diet rich in fruits and vegetables as an intervention in women only, since the data appear to be more compelling in that gender group. Also, more research into the area of gender differences in carcinogen metabolism and how that might be modulated by diet should also be pursued. Finally, although it appears obvious, smoking cessation programs targeted specifically toward women smokers, as well as nonsmoking women married to smokers, would also address much of the causation of women's lung cancers.

6. Colorectal Cancer

The genetics of colorectal cancer, although well defined and delineated as to where and when specific mutations participate in the carcinogenesis process, can account for only about 10–15% of cancers. That leaves over 85% which are considered to be nonfamilial and which may have a significant dietary etiology in both men and women.

However, the hormonal environment for women is quite different from that of men, and as such, we see an intriguing impact of female reproductive factors on colorectal cancer in women. It would appear that some of the factors which influence risk for breast cancer, such as early pregnancy and later menarche, may also decrease risk for colon cancer in women. However, exogenous hormone use, either as oral contraceptives or estrogen replacement therapy, has been seen in some studies to be protective and in others as risk-enhancing. Interestingly, the most recent studies published appear to definitely support the hypothesis that HRT in postmenopausal women lowers their risk of colorectal cancer.

Long-term use of tobacco and alcohol consumption have been linked to many cancers, among them colorectal cancer. The long induction period for colorectal cancer associated with tobacco use has allowed the connection in women to finally emerge. As for alcoholic beverage consumption, a small number of studies have been done in women and have not demonstrated strong associations between alcohol and colorectal cancer or polyps, although the Nurses' Health Study cohort has shown an elevated risk. Nonsteroidal anti-inflammatory drug use in women has been shown to somewhat reduce colorectal cancer risk, with nonaspirin compounds appearing to confer greater protection.

The scientific literature has been absolutely inundated during the past 20 years with studies of dietary factors and risk for colorectal cancer. However, only a small number of these studies have separated the results by gender, and only a very few of them have examined the influence of dietary intake in women alone. In general, for both males and females, there is increased risk associated with a large body mass index, low levels of physical activity, and high energy intake.

When examining the role of specific nutrients in colorectal cancer in women, there appears to emerge a puzzling dichotomy between the results of the only two prospective cohort studies in women, the Nurses' Health Study and the Iowa Women's Health Study. Although both cohort studies used the same dietary assessment questionnaire, the results obtained for a number of dietary factors were not similar. For dietary fat and red meat, there was a direct association with colon cancer risk in the Nurses' Study and a null association in the Iowa Study. For dairy foods, calcium, and vitamin D intakes, there was no association in the Nurses' Study and a nonsignificant decrease after multivariate adjustment in the Iowa Study. However, in two smaller studies, an analysis of Utah women showed a halving of risk and nearly that same decrease was also seen in an Australian study. For antioxidant vitamins, the Iowa Study found total vitamin E intake to be inversely associated with risk for colorectal cancer, which seemed to decrease with age, whereas there was no association seen in the Nurses' Health Study.

The influence of increased fruit and vegetable consumption on colorectal cancer risk in women was analyzed in the Iowa Women's Health Study, and a decrease in risk was found. In the Nurses' Health Study, only vegetable and fruit fiber intakes were analyzed; only fiber from fruit was associated with any appreciable reduction in risk, and the overall trend did not attain statistical significance. Thus, we see that the most compelling dietary recommendation that can be made for colorectal cancer prevention appears to be to consume more fruits and vegetables and reduce overall fat intake.

C. American Cancer Society Nutrition Guidelines

The American Cancer Society (ACS) publishes nutrition guidelines to advise the public about dietary practices that may reduce cancer.[4] According to their statistics, the scientific evidence suggests that one-third of the annual 500,000 cancer deaths in the United States each year are due to dietary factors, with another one-third attributable to cigarette smoking. However, for the majority of Americans who do not smoke cigarettes, dietary choices become the most important modifiable determinants of cancer risk.[5] The ACS advisory panel also concluded that although genetics is a significant factor in the development of cancer, most cancers cannot be explained by hereditary factors alone. Recently, the ACS 1996 Advisory Committee on Diet, Nutrition, and Cancer met and reaffirmed its recommendations for reducing the risk of cancer in Americans. The guidelines include the following:[4]

1. Choose most of the foods you eat from plant sources.
2. Limit your intake of high-fat foods, particularly from animal sources.
3. Be physically active: achieve and maintain a healthy weight.
4. Limit consumption of alcoholic beverages, if you drink at all.

The scientific evidence for these recommendations is quite strong for cancers of many sites. Specific to those cancers in women discussed in this book, there is strong evidence that increased consumption of vegetables reduces the risk of colorectal cancer, as well as lung cancer. We all know that the major risk for lung cancer is smoking cigarettes, but diet appears to also modify that risk. The risk of high-fat diets has been associated with colorectal cancer in women, although the association between high-fat diets and breast cancer is much weaker. Physical activity can protect against some cancers, especially when there is an imbalance in caloric intake leading to overweight and obesity, both of which have been linked to cancers of the colon and endometrium and of the breast in postmenopausal women.[4] The final guideline about limiting consumption of alcoholic beverages may be most relevant to breast cancer among cancers in women, in that there appears to be a weak association between alcohol intake and risk for breast cancer. However, the

ACS guidelines on alcohol are specifically targeted more to prevention of oral and esophageal cancers, which are more prevalent in men. The cardiovascular benefits of a moderate intake of alcoholic beverages may outweigh the risk of cancer in men older than 50 years and in women older than 60.[4] However, the ACS still recommends that women with an unusually high risk of breast cancer consider total abstinence from alcohol.[4] However, based upon our review of the literature, we are of the opinion that this may be a premature recommendation.

II. DIRECTIONS FOR FUTURE RESEARCH

A. Genetics

In this book we have briefly reviewed the genetics associated with the six major cancer sites in women. The genetic contribution to cancer etiology has been best described for colorectal, breast, and ovarian cancer. But the caveat here is that even with the genetics so carefully defined in the case of those cancers, the hereditary forms of these cancers still only represent about 5–15% of all the cases that occur. This leaves the overwhelming number of incident cancers each year in the category of no apparent genetic basis at all, except for the occurrence of somatic mutations in the generalizable cancer-related genes, such as tumor suppressor genes and other oncogenes. It is the opinion of these authors that a future direction for research would be into how diet and nutrition act to protect against these specific mutations which appear to hasten the carcinogenic process in high-risk populations.

B. Biomarkers

One of the important tools of cancer research is the preneoplastic lesion, a surrogate endpoint, or a biomarker of the neoplastic process that is evident long before the tumor appears. These harbingers of cancer are extremely important in the research into how diet and nutrition interventions might prevent the cancer development process. Unfortunately, there are no reliable and predictive biomarkers for most cancers in women, with the exception of the abnormal Pap smear and the colorectal polyp. For ovarian, endometrial, and lung cancers, there is a serious lack of any early identifiable marker of the neoplastic process in these tissues. For breast tissue, the earliest lesion that can be recognized is ductal carcinoma *in situ*, which is already considered a cancerous lesion.[6] Research into prevention of these cancers should focus on the development of tissue, radiographic, or some other reliable marker for an impending cancer, so that intervention studies may be conducted and attempts made to modulate the biomarker and potentially the cancer risk itself.

C. Cancer Prevention Strategies for Cervical, Endometrial, and Ovarian Cancers

A number of cancer chemoprevention strategies for cervical, endometrial, and ovarian cancers are being considered.[7] The role for nutritional chemoprevention is greatest for cervical cancer in that there are several potentially effective agents, including folic acid, beta-carotene, and vitamin C. A suitable cohort would be patients with cervical intraepithelial neoplasia (CIN) II and III, which could be used as a biomarker. In fact, Phase II and Phase III chemoprevention trials of beta-carotene in CIN II and III and vitamin C alone and combined with beta-carotene in CIN II are ongoing.[7] Vaccination against HPV infection is also another considered preventive strategy, although it is independent of nutritional factors.

In the endometrium and ovary, fewer cancer chemopreventive strategies have emerged, except for the use of antiestrogens and progestins.[7] A potential cohort with a biomarker for risk would be patients with atypical hyperplasia of the uterine corpus. However, for these patients, the cancer prevention strategy would be hormonal, not nutritionally based. Except for the ACS recommendation of avoiding obesity and pursuing a lower fat diet, nothing specific is available for targeted dietary prevention of this cancer.

Women who are at high risk for ovarian cancer may benefit from taking oral contraceptives to reduce ovulation frequency.[7] There are no biomarkers in the ovary that would allow women to participate in Phase II cancer prevention trials; however, it is of interest that a Phase III trial of the retinoid fenretinamide in breast cancer patients found a reduced ovarian cancer incidence in those taking the drug compared to the placebo.[7] Thus, retinoids may have a potential chemopreventive action against ovarian cancer, but this does not suggest that there are now available dietary means that could be preventive.

D. Conclusions

In summary, when the evidence is completely assessed for nutritional influences on women's cancers, the major theme that emerges is the interaction of nutritional status with a hormonal environment that is unique to females. This hormonal overlay appears to be a key player in all the major cancers in women, even down to their differential susceptibility to colorectal and lung cancers. This is a fact of life and is immutable. What we can change is the general opinion that gender does not impact environmental susceptibility. For this reason, it is important that we move toward a direction in the future that separately assesses the sexes in epidemiologic studies and intervention trials and that we focus research on the causes of human cancer within the hormonal framework that we find inescapable. Now that women's health issues have come into national prominence, the entire field of nutritional epidemiology of cancer may have to develop a new gender-specific perspective.

REFERENCES

1. ·Department of Health and Human Services, Public Health Service, *Healthy People 2000*, Jones and Bartlett Publishers, Boston, 1992, chap. 16.
2. Klein, R., *Healthy People 2000* review: women's cancers, *J. Natl. Cancer Inst.*, 88, 1427, 1996.
3. Colditz, G.A. and Frazier, A.L., Models of breast cancer show that risk is set by events of early life: prevention efforts must shift focus, *Cancer Epidemiol. Biomarkers Prev.*, 4, 567, 1995.
4. American Cancer Society 1996 Advisory Committee on Diet, Nutrition, and Cancer Prevention, Guidelines on diet, nutrition, and cancer prevention: reducing the risk of cancer with healthy food choices and physical activity, *CA Cancer J. Clin.*, 46, 325, 1996.
5. McGinnis, J.M. and Foege, W.H., Actual causes of death in the United States, *J. Am. Med. Assoc.*, 270, 2207, 1993.
6. Dhinga, K., A Phase II chemoprevention trial to identify surrogate endpoint biomarkers in breast cancer, *J. Cell. Biochem.*, 23, 19, 1995.
7. Kelloff, G.J., Boone, C.W., Crowell, J.A., Nayfield, S.G., Hawk, E., Steele, V.E., Lubet, R.A., and Sigman, C.C., Strategies for Phase II cancer chemoprevention trials: cervix, endometrium, and ovary, *J. Cell. Biochem.*, 23, 1, 1995.

INDEX